A Natural History of Homosexuality

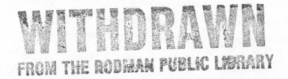

A NATURAL HISTORY OF
Homosexuality

Francis Mark Mondimore 1953

THE JOHNS HOPKINS UNIVERSITY PRESS
BALTIMORE AND LONDON

The Johns Hopkins University Press
2715 North Charles Street
Baltimore, Maryland 21218-4319
The Johns Hopkins Press Ltd., London

Library of Congress Cataloging-in-Publication Data will be found
at the end of this book.

A catalog record for this book is available from the British Library.

ISBN 0-8018-5349-4
ISBN 0-8018-5440-7 (pbk.)

Illustrations on pages 110, 115, 124, and 152 by Jacqueline Schaffer.

There is a principle which is a bar against all information, which is proof against all arguments and which cannot fail to keep a man in everlasting ignorance—that principle is contempt prior to investigation.

HERBERT SPENCER

Contents

Preface

I hope you will find *A Natural History of Homosexuality* an easy-to-understand, noncontroversial introductory book on a complex and frequently controversial subject. I must admit that when my editor first suggested calling this book a "natural history," I had my doubts. But when she read the definition of "natural history" to me over the phone, I realized that this was indeed an apt description of the book I had written. A "natural history" is, after all, "the study and description of organisms and natural objects, their origins, evolution and interrelationships" (*The American Heritage Dictionary of the English Language*, 1992).

Despite the availability of many books about homosexuality for psychologists, psychiatrists, counselors, and behavioral scientists, few have been written for the nonscientific audience which address the subject in any depth. Small wonder—as I discovered—for the scientific literature on the subject is intricate and subtle. Although newspapers seem to report on discoveries of brain centers and genes linked to homosexuality every couple of months, readers without a scientific background who want more information on these discoveries may find themselves befuddled when they turn to the scientific works on the topic, overwhelmed by its complexity and ultimately confused about conclusions.

More accessible and easier-to-read books about homosexuality often concentrate on the personal experience of coming to terms with homosexuality and tend to treat the more scientific aspects of the study of sexual orientation in a superficial way. They can leave questions about the biology, genetics, and psychology of homosexuality unanswered.

In this book I hope to bridge this gap, providing an introduction to available knowledge on homosexuality from a variety of viewpoints for the general reader. What are some of the questions I hope to address?

"Why am I gay/lesbian?" is a question many individuals seek to answer at some point in their lives. A local coordinator of the national organization P-FLAG (Parents and Families and Friends of Lesbians and Gays) told me that its membership is "hungry" for answers to the question "Why is my child gay/lesbian?" We take for granted that there is a biology of gender—males and females differ in anatomy and physiology. Is there also a biology of sexual orientation? Several researchers have reported discovering brain structures that seem to be different in heterosexual and homosexual individuals. What do these studies mean?

What is the process by which individuals come to think of themselves as homosexual? Many (though certainly not all) people who discover homosexual feelings within themselves are at first bewildered and ashamed of these feelings. How do gay people come to accept and celebrate their sexual identity? And why is it that some do not? Is the process the same in other cultures? Has it always been the same? What were the historical events that shaped our thinking about homosexuality?

Where does bisexuality fit in? How about transsexualism (the phenomenon of feeling like a "woman trapped in a man's body" or vice versa)? What, if anything, do these have to do with homosexuality?

"Gay rights" was a significant issue in the 1992 presidential election. Several states have recently held referenda to amend their constitutions to prevent homosexuals from ever being recognized as a minority group. What is it about homosexuality which would justify changing a state constitution? Why do these issues cause so much conflict in our society? Have there been other times or other cultures in which they did not?

Many employers now provide insurance benefits to the partners of gay and lesbian employees. Others (including the American Armed

Forces) have waged court battles to retain their prerogative to terminate homosexual employees because of their private sexual behavior. Consensual sexual contact between members of the same sex is a crime in some states—but discrimination against individuals based on sexual orientation is a crime in others. Conservative political groups protest government funding for artworks that they claim "promote homosexuality," but openly homosexual musicians, singers, and actors draw hundreds of thousands to their performances, and plays and films with gay and lesbian characters have been big box office hits. Many large religious denominations in the United States preach tolerance and acceptance of homosexuals, but even the most liberal congregations struggle with whether to allow gay and lesbian clergy to be ordained and whether to bless the partnerships of gay and lesbian couples with marriage ceremonies. Why do our attitudes so persistently elude consensus and consistency? Is there relevant scientific information that can inform these discussions and point toward logical, fair, and moral laws and policies?

It became clear early on in the writing of this book that to accomplish the ambitious goal of introducing people to the information they needed to understand homosexuality would mean covering quite a bit of ground. I had originally thought to write a short explanatory work on an aspect of homosexuality with which I, a psychiatrist with a background in biology, was most familiar and found the most interesting—the biology of sexual orientation. Simon LeVay's study demonstrating brain differences between homosexual and heterosexual men had appeared and soon was joined by other studies on biological factors in homosexuality, like those on "gay genes." It might be argued that the most important new information on homosexuality—but the most difficult for the layperson to grasp—is this new work on the neurology and genetics of sexual orientation.

It quickly became apparent to me, however, that a discussion of biology wouldn't shed much light on the questions I've posed in preceding paragraphs. The biology of sexuality may be interesting, but it provides only one perspective from which to view this complex subject. And perhaps more than any other topic, sexuality needs to be examined from many perspectives in order to be understood. What are some of these perspectives?

Since the word *homosexuality* was coined in 1869, many scientists in a variety of fields have sought to understand it better:

- Neuroscientists and physiologists have examined the biological basis of sexual behaviors by investigating the functioning of the brain and nervous system, sexual anatomy, and the regulation of hormonal systems in humans and animals.
- Behavioral scientists have concerned themselves with the development of a homosexual identity, a process starting in preadolescence and continuing into adulthood and indeed throughout an individual's lifetime.
- Psychologists and psychiatrists have explored the "antecedents" of adult sexuality in children and even infants.
- Sociologists and anthropologists have examined the social context of homosexuality. Some have argued that society shapes—even constructs—the homosexual identity.
- Historians have examined the historical contexts and events that have shaped our thinking and attitudes about homosexuality.
- Zoologists have examined same-sex behavior in animals as a model for human homosexuality.
- Evolutionary biologists have theorized about the genetics and even evolution of homosexuality.

It is a daunting task to bridge the discontinuities among these fields and bring together their often divergent points of view into a unified picture. But if I've accomplished my goal, a coherent, if complex, picture will emerge which points to some conclusions that are not difficult to understand. One of these conclusions is that homosexuality is a human condition that develops as do most other complex behavioral phenomena, through a complicated and quite distinctly human intermingling of many factors—biological, psychological, and social. It will also become clear that any understanding based too much on only one of these factors is simply incomplete.

My research on the history of attitudes and theories about homosexuality has been the most rewarding and one of the most enjoyable aspects of writing this book. I believe that there is no better way to understand something than to examine it from a historical perspective. The story is incomplete without meeting the likes of Anne Lister, Oscar Wilde, and Harry Hay and seeing how events like the trial of the Knights Templar in 1307, the Nazi Holocaust, and the beginnings of the AIDS epidemic have affected our thinking about homosexuality, not to mention the lives of gays and lesbians—then and now.

Inevitably, the exploration of a topic of such complexity in a single volume requires simplifying ideas and condensing information. A whole book could be written about some aspects of homosexuality which are covered here in only a few pages. (In many instances, a good book *has* been written—and is included in the reading list in the back of the book.) Since I want this to be an introductory book for those who don't know where to begin, frequently I have laid out only the basic outlines of complex ideas and then listed the "next step" works in the endnotes for those who are interested in learning more.

Some may wish to criticize what might appear to be an emphasis on "causes" of homosexuality. The very word *cause* conjures up the implication that homosexuality is a disease state whose deviation from "normal" demands explanation. At a national meeting I attended some years back on gay and lesbian health issues, scientists presenting results of their work on genetics and brain structure were harshly criticized by some in the audience who charged that "treatment" and even prevention of homosexuality were the goals of such work. Indeed, many scientists have had exactly these goals in mind as they investigated various aspects of homosexuality.

The psychiatric literature, for example, is full of papers and books in which the assumption that homosexuality is a mental illness is stated quite clearly—an assumption that is not based on very good science. Good science gathers information and seeks to explain and understand it, avoiding preconceptions as much as possible. Good science does not prejudge what is normal or abnormal; it merely assembles information logically and postulates how different pieces of information might be related to each other. In the field of human sexuality, good science is exemplified by the work that Alfred Kinsey and his co-workers did in the 1940s. Kinsey made no assumptions about what was normal or abnormal but set out simply to discover what *is* in the realm of human sexual behavior. His findings—that homosexuality is commonplace and that gay and lesbian people form a significant proportion of the population—resounded like a thunderclap throughout the psychological and psychiatric community. Most behavioral scientists rejected his data and reviled him personally for his conclusions. Methodological error casts some doubt on the precision of Kinsey's numbers, but *Sexual Behavior in the Human Male* remains a watershed work, and no exploration of sexual orientation can be written which does not refer to it. Kinsey's results were enthusiastically received by budding gay and lesbian rights organizations, energizing their efforts to define gay people as an oppressed minority rather than a collection of deviants.

History shows that it has been the bigoted and judgmental who have resisted the gathering of scientific data on homosexuality. One of the first and largest libraries of case studies and other material for the study of sexual behavior, the Institute of Sexual Science of the German psychiatrist Magnus Hirschfeld, was looted and burned by the Nazis in 1933. Hirschfeld was another pioneer who preached understanding and acceptance of homosexuals and who sought to support his activism by scientific methods. His success in gaining the attention of influential German social scientists, physicians, and politicians with careful and sound scientific inquiry was what made him so threatening to the Nazis.

It is my hope that those who have misgivings about scientific probes into the biological underpinnings of homosexuality will be gratified, as I have been, to learn that far from reinforcing the disease model, good scientific work points toward a very humanistic model that sees homosexuality as a normative variation of human sexual behavior.

Acknowledgments

The author wishes to thank those who contributed to this project. Thanks to Lynn Kellen and Larry Tilson, for their thorough and thoughtful analysis of the manuscript and for their valuable criticism and excellent suggestions. Thanks to Dr. Pleas Geyer, for sharing his expertise on Sigmund Freud and psychoanalysis.

Thanks to Jacqueline Schaffer, for her lucid illustrations, and to Mr. Merlin Holland, for permission to reproduce the photograph of Oscar Wilde and Alfred Douglas.

Special thanks to all the wonderful people at the Johns Hopkins University Press, most especially my editor, Jacqueline Wehmueller, not only for her superb editorial advice and assistance but also for being an inexhaustible source of encouragement when the going got rough.

And of course, thanks to my partner, Jay Allen Rubin, for being there whenever I needed him and also for (usually) knowing when this sometimes cranky writer was better left alone.

PART I

Sexual Histories

I was surprised not too long ago to hear a friend remark that his six-year-old didn't know what a record was. Helping his father clean out their attic and coming across his dad's vinyl rock and roll collection, my friend's son, who was familiar only with compact disc recordings, had to be told that these dull black platters were the nearly obsolete precursors to the iridescent CDs he knew well. Not too long ago, buying a music recording required choosing between two alternative recording technologies: vinyl 33⅓ rpm record albums or compact discs. Now, apparently, a whole new generation of music recording buyers are browsing racks of CDs at music stores all over the country oblivious to the fact that what seems to them the only existing category of recording was considered a high-tech curiosity only fifteen or so years ago.

My friend's story recalled another discussion about musical categories, one that I had heard on the radio years ago, in which a classical guitarist lamented having repeatedly to identify his instrument to young people as an "*acoustic* guitar." After the invention of the electric guitar in the 1950s, it had become necessary to devise a label for guitars that were not electric. Where there had been only one category, there were now two. At one time, he could have simply said that he played the guitar; now further categorization was needed, to communicate which of two instruments, each with a vastly different sound and performance style, he played.

Categories are abstract concepts by which we attempt to capture the essences of the things we categorize. Categorizing something implies that it shares a set of attributes with all the other things that are in the same category and that is different in some way from things in other categories. Categories help us make sense of the world. As technology advances, or as we learn more about the essences of what we are attempting to classify, new categories are created and old ones abandoned.

Nowhere is this shifting of categories over time more evident than in the attempt to categorize people and behavior, most especially sexual behavior. One of the first problems encountered when one attempts to examine sexual behavior is that categories we may take for granted, for example, the categories "homosexual" and "heterosexual," have fuzzy borders and overlapping territories. There are even more problems when we try to apply *our* categories to persons in cultures different from our own. In ancient cultures and remote preindustrial societies, our categories seem irrelevant. Qualities that we consider to be the "essences" of persons as sexual creatures other societies find almost inconsequential. One can't hope to understand homosexuality without defining the category, and contrary to what you may have read in dictionaries and textbooks, defining homosexuality is a fiendishly difficult task. This is especially true if you attempt to come up with a definition that fits not only twentieth-century Americans and Europeans but also peoples in other places and times. This is, in fact, nearly impossible, as we'll see in Chapter 1. What becomes clear as one looks at other times and other cultures is that there have been *many* definitions of homosexuality—and I think that each of these definitions has something valuable to teach us.

Over the last thousand years or so people have defined homosexuality as a sexual preference (like a preference for white wine rather than red), as a gift from the gods bestowing great wisdom and powers of healing, as a terrible sin, as a mental illness, as a natural human variation. In this section, we will explore the ways of understanding and defining homosexuality which have developed from ancient times until the present. There have been—and still are—many answers to the question "What is homosexuality?" A historical perspective is crucial to understanding homosexuality as it exists today in our society—and also gives me the opportunity to tell some terrific stories about exotic places and fascinating people.

ONE

Before Homosexuality

Observations from Other Cultures

The word *homosexuality* did not exist prior to 1869, when it appeared in a pamphlet that took the form of an open letter to the German minister of justice (the German word is *homosexualität*). A new penal code for the North German Federation was being drafted, and a debate had arisen over whether to retain the section of the Prussian criminal code which made sexual contact between persons of the same gender a crime. The pamphlet's author, Karl Maria Kertbeny (1824–82), was one of several writers and jurists who were beginning to develop the concept of sexual orientation. This idea—that some individuals' sexual attraction for persons of the same sex was an inherent and unchanging aspect of their personality—was radically new. Thousands of years of recorded history and the rise and fall of sophisticated and complex societies occurred *before homosexuality* existed as a word or even as an idea. In order to understand homosexuality today, we need to understand how same-sex eroticism fit into these ancient cultures.

The ancient Greek and Latin languages have no word that can be translated as *homosexual*, largely because these societies did not have the same sexual categories that we do. Our concepts and categories of sexual expression are based on the genders of the two partners involved: *heterosexuality* when the partners are of the opposite sex, and *homosexuality* when the partners are of the same sex. In other times and among other peoples, this way of thinking about people simply doesn't seem to apply—anthropologists, historians, and sociologists have described many cultures in which same-sex eroticism occupies a very different place than it does in our own. Anthropologist Margaret Mead had this diversity in mind when she stated in 1935 that "when we study the simpler societies, we cannot but be impressed with the many ways in which man has taken a few hints and woven them into the beautiful imaginative social fabrics that we call civilizations."[1] Just as the Greeks and Romans had no words for our sexual categories, the Native American societies described by explorers, missionaries, and anthropologists from the seventeenth century onward had sexual categories for which *we* have no words.

Consequently, in the sections that follow—an exploration of attitudes and customs of ancient peoples toward same-sex eroticism—the modern concepts of "homosexuality" or "sexual orientation" will be conspicuous by their absence. Within these cultures, sexual contact between persons of the same sex is not necessarily seen as characteristic of a particular group or subset of persons; there is no category for "homosexuals." On the contrary, in some cultures, same-sex eroticism was an expected part of the sexual experience of every member of society, which would seem to argue against the existence of "homosexuality" as a personal attribute at all.

Ancient Greece

Victorian British classicists were terribly embarrassed by references in the works of Plato and other Greek philosophers to sexual relationships between men. In a passage in E. M. Forster's autobiographical novel *Maurice*, written at the turn of the nineteenth century about the awakening of homoerotic feelings in an Oxford undergraduate, a student translating a section of a philosophical work is instructed by the professor to "omit a reference to the unspeakable vice of the Greeks."[2] Translations of various works of Greek philosophy were sanitized to eliminate references to erotic feelings of adult men for younger men.

In more modern translations, these passages are unambiguously homoerotic:

> "What do you think of the young man, Socrates?" said Khairephon.
> "Doesn't he have a handsome face?"

"Marvelously so!" I said.

"Well," he said, "if he'd only take his cloak off, you'd forget he has a face at all, he's so overwhelmingly beautiful to look at."[3]

An extensive discussion of the origins, meaning, and philosophy of love occurs in Plato's *Symposium*, thought to have been written about 386 B.C. In one section, several participants ponder the relative merits of several different types of love. Phaedrus describes the mythical Orpheus, who entered the Underworld to rescue his wife from the realm of the dead, and also Achilles, the Greek warrior of Homer's epic *Iliad*, killed while attempting to revenge the death of his warrior lover Patroclus. Orpheus is punished for the cowardly behavior that made him fail in his mission, while Achilles is "sent to the Islands of the Blest" for his valor.

Further along in *Symposium*, a young man named Alkibiades, who has arrived for the philosophical gathering late (and drunk), describes his attempts to seduce the great philosopher Socrates—in a narrative that could have come right out of the pages of contemporary gay fiction. "Now, I fancied that he was seriously enamored of my beauty," Alkibiades begins, and he goes on to describe how he discreetly but relentlessly contrives increasingly irresistible opportunities for the philosopher to be intimate with him. Alkibiades begins by arranging solitary meetings, but Socrates is cool. Even wrestling matches at the gymnasium fail to arouse him. Alkibiades invites Socrates to dinner, but his distinguished guest leaves immediately after the meal. A second dinner at first seems to be more promising: "After we had supped, I went on conversing far into the night, and when he wanted to go away, I pretended that the hour was late and that he had much better remain." Socrates falls asleep, but Alkibiades shakes him awake and says, "Of all the lovers I have ever had, you are the only one who is worthy of me." Socrates replies with an irony that is lost on the hot-blooded young man, who nevertheless climbs into bed with the philosopher: "And there I lay during the whole night having this wonderful monster in my arms." Alkibiades, convinced that his machinations have finally paid off, is astounded that Socrates falls off to sleep again and is mortified to have to report that nothing more happened: "In the morning, when I awoke, I arose from the couch of a father or an elder brother."[4]

The narrative, especially Socrates' lack of interest in Alkibiades, spurs further discussion among the philosophers present about the types and qualities of love, and Socrates' restraint and self-control is admired by all. The important point for the purposes of this discussion is Plato's implication that Socrates did not react to Alkibiades' solicitations as expected—as many men would have. To have spent time alone with, wrestled with, eaten dinner alone with, and even spent the night in the bed of an attractive, intelligent young man and allow "nothing" to happen is presented as a surprising turn of events.

Numerous artistic and literary works from this period depict male homosexuality. The book *Greek Homosexuality*, by classical scholar K. J. Dover, devotes twenty pages to a list of vases and other pieces of pottery dating from the fourth and fifth centuries B.C. which have homoerotic decorations. Greek theater pieces have numerous allusions to sexual contact between men. Cyclops, a character in Euripides' *The Cyclops*, baldly proclaims, "I prefer boys to girls."[5]

These men were not homosexual—not in the modern meaning of that term. The Greeks had no such word or concept. It is perhaps more correct to say that the Greeks practiced a sort of "bisexuality" in that, for men at least, sexual activity with partners of both sexes was

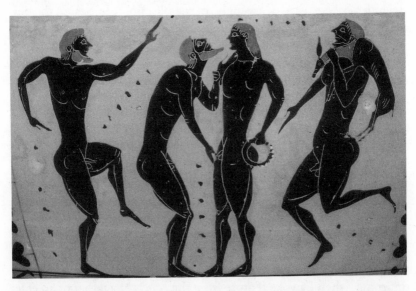

An image from a Greek vase showing an *erastes* and an *eromenos*, sixth century B.C. (Courtesy of the Foto Museum, Staatliche Antikensammlungen und Glyptothek, Munich)

accepted. Even this term fails to describe Greek sexuality accurately because fundamental differences between the sexual mores of ancient Greece and those of our society make comparisons between the cultures difficult. Exploring Greek sexual mores a bit further and comparing them with our own will illustrate these differences.

In the late twentieth century, the highest expression of sexuality is usually considered to be in the setting of a committed, caring relationship between two persons based on mutual respect and resulting from free choice. Romantic love is praised and treasured, seen as a prelude to a deeper bonding process, which leads to the "happily ever after" most of us wish for. This paired relationship forms the foundation for procreation, child rearing, and family relationships in our culture; romantic love leads to marriage, which leads to sexuality and procreation. Examination of the ancient Greek society reveals that sexuality and procreation were not linked in the same way. Sex was necessary, and marriage the only legitimate setting, for procreation, but sexual pleasure was available, for men at least, in a variety of forms outside marriage as well. Since the concept of romantic love had yet to develop fully, a man did not have to be sexually faithful within marriage to remain honorable. (The rules were quite different for women, as we will see.)

Although sexual pleasure and marriage were not necessarily linked, sexuality and domination most certainly were. Far from being a mutual experience, sexual activity always had a directional quality for the Greeks. Sex was something one "did" to someone, and anatomic imperative dictated that it was the man (or more precisely the penis) that did the doing. Even the language of sexuality in the two cultures reflects this difference in attitude. The Greeks had specific words to describe various sexual activities, often specifying a particular pairing of penis and orifice (such as *paedico*, which means "to penetrate anally"). In modern English the accepted words and phrases used to describe sexual contact convey the mutuality and reciprocity that our culture expects of legitimate and respected kinds of sexuality: people "make love," "have sex," and "have intercourse." More "directional" words, which convey domination, are still around but are considered obscene or crude: to "screw" or "fuck" someone, or to "get laid."

Conceptualizing sexual acts exclusively in terms of domination and submission provided a basis for the practice of humiliating conquered enemies—male and female—by raping them. To be penetrated unwillingly was shameful and degrading. The social acceptability of a sexual act was not determined by the gender of the partners but rather by the balance of power between them. To quote David Halperin, a classicist who has written much on the issue of Greek homosexuality: "In classical Athens, sexual objects came in two different kinds—not male and female but active and passive, aggressive and submissive."[6]

Among the ancient Greeks, sexual contact between males of the same social group was scrupulously concerned with status and was played out according to rules that assured that neither party was degraded or open to accusations of licentiousness. The idealized sexual partnership between men consisted of an active older and a passive younger partner. While the older took pleasure in the sexual act, the younger partner was expected not to. The two roles were distinguished by having different labels; the older partner was called the *erastes* and the younger the *eromenos*. There was never oral or anal contact, only intracrural intercourse, illustrated on pottery paintings as the older partner inserting his penis between the thighs of the younger as both are standing. Just how "young" the eromenos should have been has been debated. Some pottery decorations show what appear to be prepubertal males being fondled by men, and others depict tall, well-muscled, robust young adults as partners of older men. Halperin concludes from his survey of ancient Greek writings and artworks that this culture considered young men most sexually attractive in late adolescence, "in that slender zone between boyhood and manhood . . . corresponding roughly to the life-stage of American undergraduates."[7] Once the eromenos was past this stage, the relationship was expected to end. The former eromenos would now marry a woman, but he could also become an erastes, the older partner, in a new sexual relationship with a younger man.

Among the ancient Greeks, honorable and accepted sexual practices for men were not defined by the gender of one's partner or by whether sex took place within an exclusive relationship based on romantic love. Instead, whether a particular sexual pairing was considered acceptable or not depended on the age and social standing of the partner. For men at least, whether the partner was male or female and whether one was married to his partner was almost inconsequential. It was perfectly acceptable, in fact expected, that a man would have a wife and an eromenos simultaneously—at least some of the time.

The erastes/eromenos relationship was celebrated in poetry and was used to explicate the philosophy of love and beauty by Plato. Male couples decorated vases and urns used as ordinary household containers. Love for a young man was idealized as having special qualities that set it apart from the love of women, "heavenly love" as opposed to "common love," as Plato describes it in the *Symposium*.[8] Sexual relationships between males were not only tolerated but celebrated as necessary complements to procreative sex.

It is important to remember that the erastes/eromenos relationship was an idealized model for sexual contact between males and that the realities of passion may have more closely resembled the lusty comedies of Aristophanes. It is probably erroneous to assume that intracrural intercourse was the exclusive form of intimacy between males among the ancient Greeks. There are vase depictions of and written references to anal intercourse, and one can assume that intracrural intercourse was the exception rather than the rule in the male brothels. But since the penetrated man was considered to be taking the passive role of a woman and essentially abdicating the valued masculine role, the passive role was devalued, and passive partners were lampooned in the Greek comedies. The refined dialogues of Plato may not reflect the true breadth of Greek sexuality any more than the plays of George Bernard Shaw reflect that of Victorian England.

Although Greek writings depict women and young men as almost interchangeable objects of sexual desire for many men, the Greeks recognized that some men were preferentially attracted to other men throughout their lives. Again separating sexual pleasure from sexual duty, these men would marry and would father children, but they still sought young men as preferred sexual partners. The philosophers Bion and Zeno as well as Alexander the Great were known for their almost exclusive interest in men.[9]

Aristophanes explains these variations in sexual desires by giving an account of powerful mythological human ancestors who had two heads, two sets of arms and legs—and two sets of sexual organs. Some of these creatures were half male and half female, but others were double males and double females. Robust and proud, these creatures tried to climb into heaven and attack the gods, prompting Zeus to make them weaker by splitting them "as you slice hard boiled eggs with a hair." Each new "half" sought out its mate, male or female, same or opposite sex, depending upon the makeup of the original double creature. If descended from a "double man," "such a person is always inclined to be an erastes or an eromenos, as he always welcomes what is akin. So when one of these meets his own proper half . . . then they are wonderfully overwhelmed with affection and intimacy and love, and never wish to be apart for a moment." Aristophanes goes on to say that such men "naturally do not trouble about marriage and getting a family but that law and custom compels them."[10] Striking by its absence is the lack of a label for such a person. Although the explanatory myth of Aristophanes comes very close to being an attempt to describe the origins of sexual orientation in its modern sense, the storyteller felt no compulsion to affix labels to his categories. The Greeks had no words for homosexuality or heterosexuality because all men were assumed to be capable of passionate feelings for attractive men as well as for women. These attitudes are inextricably linked to the male domination of Greek society and to a domination/submission model for sexual relations; there was no criticism of a male who sexually dominated anyone, male or female.

Although the modern term for female homosexuality takes its name from that of the Greek island of Lesbos, almost nothing is known about Sappho, the island's most famous resident, who lived there during the sixth century B.C. Sappho's poetry inspired Plato to call her the tenth Muse, but the facts of her life are incomplete and derived from often conflicting secondary sources. Although most of her poems are fragmentary, among them are lyric pieces that are clearly passionate love poems addressed to women. Unfortunately, the Greeks did not record much about the sexuality of women—whether in Sappho's time or in Plato's time. In a group of choral odes of the (male) poet Alcman from the seventh century B.C., girls praise the beauty of favorite agemates,[11] and there are a few other fragments of pottery illustrations and poems. Much of what has survived, especially from later periods, is frankly pornographic. Female homoeroticism among prostitutes is depicted on vase paintings, and Greek writings from the first century A.D. begin to mention "tribadism."[12] Both the Greeks and the Romans described the tribade as a woman who either sexually penetrated other women with an artificial phallus or was imagined to possess a clitoris large enough to do so. The term *tribadism* persisted well into the twentieth century as a pejorative label for female homosexuality, although the more literary term *lesbianism* became common by the late nineteenth century.

The attitudes of the ancient Greeks toward female homosexuality simply cannot be discussed with any certainty. At least one review of the life and works of Sappho insists, however, that like their male counterparts, the women of ancient Greece, at least on Lesbos in the sixth century B.C., could express heterosexual or homosexual eroticism freely and without societal condemnation and without any need for a label: "Sappho was a poet who loved women. She was not a lesbian who wrote poetry."[13]

The Berdache Phenomenon

In their travels through North America during the mid-eighteenth century, French missionaries and explorers observed Native American men who took the roles and dress of women (*cross-gender* behaviors) and who took other men as sexual partners. The French word *berdache* (a male homosexual) was applied to these men and also to women who wore male attire and participated in hunting, warfare, and other pursuits their culture defined as masculine.[14]

The Europeans described the male berdaches as "sodomites dedicated to nefarious practices" who would "abandon themselves to the most infamous passions."[15] They were horrified to learn that cross-gender and homosexual behavior was not merely tolerated by the Indians; the berdache was respected, even revered, in some Indian groups.

Among some Native American peoples the berdache adopted the dress, mannerisms, and cultural role of the opposite sex completely. In these groups male berdaches would perform "womanly" domestic duties such as preparing food, making clothing and agricultural implements, and working the fields. Female berdaches made weapons and hunted. In other groups, the berdache kept the dress and grooming styles of his or her biological sex and assumed only the community role of the opposite sex.

Although in some groups berdaches were treated as if they were indeed of the opposite sex (for example, in some groups a male berdache was assigned the status of and was identified in ritual and taboos as a woman), in most groups they were identified as a third gender, neither man nor woman. For this reason the berdache phenomenon has been termed an example of *transgender* (*trans-*, meaning "across") *homosexuality*. For these peoples, a man who was sexually intimate with a male berdache was not really thought of as having sex with

another man. Although a biological male, the berdache was nevertheless "different" from a man—he was a biologically male person with
whom it was acceptable for a man to be sexually intimate. Female
berdaches are described in historical accounts as frequently having
"wives," or long-term female companions.[16] The berdache would not
engage in sexual relations with another berdache, this being considered taboo, a form of incest.

Berdaches were primarily homosexual—that is, they took sexual
partners of their own biological sex—but they were not exclusively so
among all peoples, and variations on the phenomenon are described in
some Indian groups. Some had sexual relations with both men and
women. Some did not adopt the berdache role until adulthood, and
some abandoned it after years of being identified as such. Some berdaches were celibate; some adopted the dress of a berdache and were
granted the status and special considerations accorded the role but
remained heterosexual in their sexual relations.

The berdache custom is thought to have been widespread in America, present in every major cultural group from the Iroquois in the
Northeast and along the eastern seaboard to the Pima, Navajo, Illinois, Arapaho, and Mohave tribes of the Great Plains; the Yanqui
and Zapotecs of Mexico; several South American tribes; and the Alas-
kan Eskimos. Portuguese explorer Pedro de Magalhales de Guandavo
found a group of female warriors as he traveled through northwest
Brazil in 1576, noting, "They wear the hair cut in the same way as men,
and go to war with bows and arrows and pursue game . . . each has a
woman to serve her, to whom she says she is married."[17] De Guandavo
named the river that flowed through the area after the female warriors
of Greek mythology: the Amazons. The American anthropologist
Ruth Underhill described the berdache status among the Papago people of the American Southwest during fieldwork done as late as the
1930s.[18]

Native American mythologies include stories of the origins of the
berdache which often form the basis of the berdache roles in Indian
culture. In the Navajo creation myth, First Man and First Woman live
in a difficult and unhappy world until they are taught farming, pottery
making, basket weaving, and the crafting of stone axes and hoes by two
twins, Turquoise Boy and White Shell Girl, the first berdaches. (The
Navajo word for berdache is *nadle*, which has been translated as "one
who is transformed.")[19] Other myths ascribe the transformation of

ordinary men and women into berdaches to supernatural intervention from animals and spirits. Several native peoples have myths in which individuals or communities are punished for trying to interfere with the "transformation." In a myth of the Mandan people, when a warrior tries to make the tribe's berdaches give up their traditional dress and special status, angry spirits punish the community and many of the people die.

The Papago people believed that children became berdaches after having supernatural dreams. Writing during the 1930s, Underhill described how parents who noticed that their son had a proclivity for women's crafts tested for the berdache gift. After placing a man's bow and arrows and a woman's basket in an enclosure of bushes and telling the boy to enter, they would set fire to the brush and observe what the boy brought with him as he ran out. If he ran out with the basket, he was proclaimed a berdache. A similar brushfire ceremony was reported by a journalist visiting California Indians in 1871.[20]

Because of his special connection with gods and spirits, the male berdache was often the group's shaman, or "medicine man." Combining the roles of priest and physician, the shaman ministered to the sick and officiated at religious ceremonies performed to ensure success in hunting and warfare and was believed to have the gift of prophecy and dream interpretation. In addition to their supernatural powers, male berdaches were honored as superior craftsmen, and their pottery and weaving skills were believed to be exceptional.

The Amazons were sometimes the most outstanding hunters and warriors of the tribe. A nineteenth-century Amazon known only as the Woman Chief of the Crow Indians of the upper Missouri is described as leading "a charmed life which, with her daring feats, elevated her to a point of honor and respect not often reached by male warriors . . . the Indians [were] proud of her, sung forth her praise in songs composed by them after each of her brave deeds. When council was held amid all the chiefs and warriors assembled, she took her place among the former, ranking third person in the band of 160 lodges."[21] This particular Amazon had not just one wife but, as was the privilege of high-ranking chiefs, three.

Just as the homosexuality of the ancient Greeks can only be understood within the context of their culture, the berdache phenomenon must be viewed in light of the culture of these ancient peoples. Two important points about them are most relevant. First, attitudes regarding sexuality were relaxed and accepting. The aboriginal Americans considered sexuality a gift from the spirit world, a pleasure to be appreciated and enjoyed freely before and during, within and outside, marriage and procreative purposes. Sexual play among children and adolescents was not forbidden or even discouraged, and homosexual bonding between male adolescents and between female adolescents was almost an expectation, although it was also expected that most would grow out of these relationships. Second, the status of women among native peoples was much more egalitarian than among their European contemporaries. Women's roles, though different from those of men, were equally valued. Women participated in tribal elections of leaders and often outnumbered men on tribal councils. Tribes were often matrilineal, individuals tracing their origins through their mother's family tree rather than their father's. Since these peoples valued the social roles of men and women equally and celebrated sexuality as a gift from the spirits, they naturally accepted diversity in gender and sexual expression.

Not all Indian groups were this accepting. Unlike most other native peoples, the Aztecs had laws punishing homosexual acts. Like adultery and incest, homosexuality was a capital offense—punishable by death. This ruthless warrior people conquered much of what is now Mexico and enforced their domination with the sacrificial murder of subject peoples. In contrast to the North American Indians, they were a militant and patrilineal society who denigrated women's social roles. It has been suggested that the Aztec law against homosexuality was an effort to deprive conquered tribes of important traditional leaders: the berdache shamans.[22]

The arrival of the conquistadors in the fifteenth century was the beginning of catastrophe and devastation for the native peoples of the New World. The Spanish conquered and attempted to rule the natives in the south, while the English and French in the north simply pushed the Indians westward. The fact that northern peoples were displaced rather than annihilated may account for the survival of North American berdache traditions long enough to be described by nineteenth- and even twentieth-century explorers and anthropologists. In Mesoamerica, however, the Spanish conquerors burned the Indian berdaches at the stake with the same zeal the Spanish Inquisitors showed in burning "sodomites" in Spain. "Sodomy" was a justification for dispossessing the Indians of their lands and wealth and was also interpreted to be the cause of the illnesses that wiped out perhaps 90 percent of the native population. In a chilling foreshadowing of attitudes seen at the beginning of the AIDS epidemic, the deaths of millions of Native Americans from measles, influenza, and smallpox, diseases spread by Europeans, were attributed to divine retribution for the sin of sodomy.

Most American native peoples understood many natural expressions of human sexuality. In cultures that stressed egalitarianism among men and women and felt connected with and respectful toward the many manifestations of the spiritual in the natural world, the berdache was valued as having a special role that neither man nor woman could fulfill.

"Homosexual" Initiation Practices

In explorations of remote areas of the world, isolated groups of people have been studied whose way of life seems not to have been touched by the complex progression of ideas which has shaped modern civilization. It is thought that these hunter-gatherer peoples in isolated areas of the Amazon, the Pacific rain forests, and remote Africa live much as they have for tens of thousands, perhaps even hundreds of thousands, of years. The study of several of these cultures by anthropologist Margaret Mead in the 1920s led to a revolutionary reappraisal of sexual attitudes, making Mead's name a household word in her time and an icon for anthropologists for years to come. More recent studies of a culture in the same area of the world have yielded information about same-sex intimacy which is just as important to the study of homosexuality.

In several primitive cultures of New Guinea, sexual relations between men and adolescent boys were an important social institution endowed with cultural and religious meanings and performing an important function in family and tribal relationships. The details of the rituals practiced by some of these tribes are jarring to modern Western sensibilities, violating one of our strictest sexual prohibitions—sexual contact between adults and prepubertal children. The study of these groups nevertheless provides a unique opportunity to observe sexual behavior in a cultural context completely different from our own. No attempt to understand homosexuality would be complete without examining these cultures, in which sexual behavior that is destructive and damaging in our culture is considered vital to the well-being of all members of this society.

The most extensive and comprehensive descriptions and accounts of a New Guinea culture that has institutionalized homosexuality have been provided by anthropologist Gilbert Herdt, who spent several years during the 1970s among a group he identifies as the Sambia people of the Papuan Eastern Highlands.[23] This area is thought to be populated by the descendants of Asian peoples who traveled by boat thirty thousand years ago to colonize the islands of New Guinea, Australia, and the thousands of other smaller islands in the South Pacific Ocean.

Central to an understanding of this culture is a familiarity with Sambian concepts of masculinity and femininity and the Sambia's beliefs about the origins of these traits in men and women. The Sambia, like many of the Melanesians, are a people who until recently were constantly engaged in warfare with the other tribes and bands with whom they share their island. Villages were decimated in intertribal raids, and the survival of the group depended directly on the battle skill of the young men. Courage and prowess in warfare were thus highly prized masculine qualities. (Although intertribal warfare was outlawed during the first part of this century when the region came to be administered by the Australian government, conflict resolution in the form of bouts of arguing and intimidation, called a "moot," is still an important and almost exclusively masculine institution.) Hunting, along with the exhausting work of clearing jungle growth for settlement and agriculture, was done by men, and strength and stamina were seen as manly virtues. Women tended the fields and bore and reared children, roles considered secondary to and merely nurturing of male-initiated functions and tasks. Among the Sambia, maleness and masculinity were greatly valued and femaleness denigrated. Women were, in fact, thought to be a dangerous threat to the masculinity of their sons and husbands, and too much female influence was thought to interfere with the development of adult masculinity. Sexual intercourse with women was considered debilitating—draining the masculine essence from the dominant male group.

Men and women were believed by the Sambia to develop adult qualities through very different mechanisms. Women were believed to be "naturally" female, their growth and development from immaturity to maturity (development of breasts, start of menstruation) occurring without any special interventions. Boys, however, were believed to require initiation rituals to become men. Male children were separated from their mothers in preadolescence (approximately age eight) to live with other young men. The Sambia believed that a boy would not mature physically and be capable of procreation himself unless he was implanted with the semen of an adult male. It was believed that all beneficial masculine qualities—strength, courage, hunting skills, and so forth—were transmitted in this way. Semen was thought of as a masculine essence without which a boy would remain small and puny. During the initiation period, pre-adolescents and adolescents underwent fasts and ritual bleeding to remove the noxious "female essences" transmitted to them by their mothers and to purify their bodies. It was believed that only by taking in the semen of an older man over a period of years would a boy come to develop secondary sexual characteristics (facial hair, the development of masculine muscle mass) as well as the psychological and temperamental characteristics of men (the aforementioned courage, aggressiveness, and so forth). As the boy matured, he took on the active role with other prepubertal males. Even after marriage, the young man lived in the "bachelor's" house for some months and was sexually intimate with both his wife and male partners.

Although the people identified as the Sambia have been the most completely studied, these types of initiation practices have been described in other groups of Melanesians throughout New Guinea. All share a common belief that the implanting of semen is essential for masculinization.

This type of institutionalized male-male sexuality has been called transgenerational homosexuality because it occurs across generations, between adults and adolescents. It has also been called sequential bisexuality,[24] referring to the fact that as he matures, each male is "homosexual" for a time and then predominantly "heterosexual" in the orientation of his sexual behavior. This form of "homosexuality" is not a stable attribute of the individual but a temporary pattern of behavior which is abandoned according to a culturally predetermined timetable. The particulars of sexual contact are also predetermined. Oral sex is practiced in some groups, anal intercourse in others. Although the sexual behavior is ritualized, it is nonetheless erotic. Herdt describes young Sambian men as "excited by it, joking among themselves about especially attractive boys whom they prefer."[25]

Herdt reports that about 5 percent of the Sambia deviated from the expected behavioral norms and describes "a few [men] who are known to have had a low interest in homosexual activities and who are extremely heterosexual; and a few who have a high interest in homosexual [activity], persisting in its practice past the appropriate time." In fact, some Sambian men are described as "homosexually oriented men" who show "an early intense interest in homosexual practices that continues into adulthood so that, as men, they enjoy, or even prefer, homosexual relationships . . . regardless of the availability of women as sex partners."[26]

Like pre-Columbian Americans, the Sambia were a hunter-gatherer people. Both groups institutionalized sexual contact between members of the same sex, but the similarities end there. Among the Sambia, homosexual contact was part of a ritual based on a primitive concept of male physiology and development. The initiation was a time-limited event, not unlike the ritual tattooing and scarring of boys to signify adulthood practiced among African tribes or Jewish ritual circumcision of male infants performed according to biblical mandates. The Sambia had no concept of a homosexual person comparable to the Indian berdache. Nevertheless, the observation that some Sambian men did not relinquish homosexual activity at the expected age suggests that a preference for same-sex eroticism characterized at least a subgroup of Sambian men. Among the Sambia, only a small minority of men seemed to become adult "homosexuals" despite universal homosexual experience during adolescence and early adult life.

More on Categories

An examination of homosexuality among ancient Greeks, pre-Columbian Native Americans, and New Guinea highlanders does not by any means completely catalogue all the cultures and societies which, unlike modern Western society, accepted, incorporated, or institutionalized homosexuality into the "mainstream" of their culture and social organization.

The ancient Romans more or less adopted Greek attitudes toward homosexuality. It is believed that pre-Roman Europeans, such as the ancient Celts, had homosexual initiation practices, and they may also have had warrior cults in which homosexual intimacy was accepted. Among ancient Mediterranean peoples, the ancient Syrians, Hittites, and Sumerians ritualized homosexual contact within religious contexts; intercourse with male temple prostitutes was part of the veneration of certain deities, comparable to the sacrifice of animals or offerings of incense. (Many biblical passages that are interpreted by some to forbid homosexuality are thought to refer instead to these idolatrous practices. See Chapter 2.)

A number of homosexual "love stories" in the mythology of many cultures suggest that egalitarian homosexuality (sexual intimacy and emotional bonding between individuals of equal social stature) was known in the ancient world. The Babylonian *Epic of Gilgamesh* describes an intimate relationship between King Gilgamesh and his warrior companion Enkidu which some interpreters regard as sexual. The biblical David describes his feelings for Jonathan by saying, "Your love to me was wonderful, surpassing the love of women" (2 Sam. 1:26).

By now it should be apparent that the word *homosexuality* refers to many, many different things. We have also seen examples of same-sex eroticism which one is hard pressed to call "homosexuality" in the modern sense. How, if at all, can these types of intimacy be related to each other? What does the ritualized transgenerational homosexuality of the Sambia have to do with the transgender homosexuality of the Indian berdache? What do either of these have to do with modern concepts of sexual orientation?

One way to make sense of this confusion about sexual categories is the so-called constructionist approach to understanding human sexuality, which holds that sexual behavior is determined by (or "constructed" from) the culture in which a person lives. In this view, no particular type of sexual behavior is any more natural or unnatural than any other. Thus, many different forms of male-male, female-female, and male-female sexuality have been observed over time and across cultures because each culture *constructs* its forms of sexuality. According to this view, sexual roles and behaviors arise out of a culture's religious, moral, and ethical beliefs, its legal traditions, politics, aesthetics, whatever scientific or traditional views of biology and psychology it may have, even factors like geography and climate. The constructionist view holds that sexual roles vary from one civilization to another because there are no innately predetermined scripts for human sexuality. What is sexually "normal" differs between the inhabitants of ancient Greece, pre-Columbian America, the New Guinea highlands, and twentieth-century industrialized countries because of inherent differences in these different cultures.

At first glance, the idea that sexual behaviors are more rooted in our culture than in our nature may seem far-fetched. But familiar examples of socially constructed sexual behaviors are not rare. In many cultures, for example, it has been quite acceptable for a man to have many wives or to have one wife and several concubines—arrangements we would find unacceptable. The voluptuous full-figured female nudes in the paintings of Peter Paul Rubens and Henri Matisse contain images of female beauty and sexual attractiveness rather different from those of popular culture today. The constructionist argument is the familiar one that beauty and sexual desire are in the eye of the beholder—but adds that the eye is always peering out through the lens of one's culture.

Contrasting with this view is that of the "essentialists," who propose that there is an innate quality in individuals, stable and unchanging over their lifetime, which drives their erotic life irresistibly toward the opposite or toward their own sex (and only rarely toward both)—whatever the cultural milieu. The essentialists argue that cultural factors may shape the expression of this personal essence but they do not *construct* it. "Essentialists" take the simultaneous existence of same-sex and opposite-sex eroticism across time and cultures as evidence for an essential human quality we have come to call sexual orientation. We will examine these two very different ways of understanding the origins of homosexuality, constructionism and essentialism, in more detail in Chapter 10.

Descriptions of the Greeks, the berdaches, and the Sambia should make us a little unsure about our categories *homosexual* and *heterosexual*—at least, they should make us think more carefully about what we mean by these words. But if we are now a little confused about categories, perhaps we can agree on a few simple facts about human sexuality: (1) same-sex eroticism has existed for thousands of years in vastly different times and cultures; (2) in some cultures, same-sex eroticism was accepted as a normal aspect of human sexuality, practiced by nearly all individuals some of the time; and (3) in nearly every culture that has been examined in any detail, a few individuals seem to experience a compelling and abiding sexual orientation toward their own sex.

❧ TWO ❧

Sodomites and Urnings

Several hundred years after the birth of Christ, Christian theologians in Europe started to examine and write about human sexuality and to develop concepts of what was moral and what was immoral, what was righteous or sinful in sexual behaviors. In A.D. 309, thirty-seven out of a set of eighty-seven canon laws enacted by the church council of Elvira (now Granada, in Spain) concerned sexual behavior—nearly half.[1] When Emperor Constantine proclaimed Christianity as the state religion of the Roman Empire a few years later, canon law would, in effect, became civil law throughout Europe. Private sexual behaviors, considered personal matters by authorities in ancient Greece and pre-Christian Rome, now became subject to ecclesiastical, and thus governmental, regulation. A newly invented word was applied to "unnatural" sexual behaviors, including what we now call homosexuality. The word was *sodomy*.

With the Enlightenment, theological authority on many matters of human behavior yielded to the methods of "natural philosophy," or what we now call the scientific method. By the mid-nineteenth century, human sexual behavior became a legitimate subject for the developing behavioral sciences to consider. It was right at this turning point that an extraordinary figure—neither theologian nor scientist—advanced startling new ideas about homosexuality and introduced another new vocabulary to express these ideas.

In this chapter, we will examine these two important sets of ideas about homosexuality. Both have had momentous impact on all theories about sexual behavior which were to follow, and both continue to influence our understanding of homosexuality even today.

Sodomites

As mentioned in the last chapter, the Greeks did not have a word for homosexuality. It was not until the early Middle Ages, when homosexual behaviors came to be defined as sins and crimes, that words were invented to identify persons who sought out sexual partners of their own gender. Condemnation of homosexuality developed as part of a shift in moral thinking about sexuality which occurred several hundred years after the birth of Jesus. This philosophy, which held that *any* form of sensuality was sinful, was derived from the writings of the Greek philosophers called the Stoics and also from some of the later writings of Plato. Writing in the third century B.C., the Stoics advocated indifference to all sources of pleasure, including, of course, sexual pleasure, and advised renunciation of any and all excessive emotions. The writings of the Stoics, rediscovered several centuries after the birth of Christ, influenced several medieval theologians, who began to advocate the idea that all sexual pleasure is sinful. The Stoics also put forth in their writings the idea that the only "natural" sexuality is intercourse for the purpose of procreation. (According to some, even procreative sex could be contaminated by too much physical pleasure and thus become sinful.) Any sexual activity that would not result in conception was considered illegitimate and "unnatural." Gradually, various disapproved sexual acts came collectively to be called *sodomy*. The word comes, of course, from the name of one of the two cities destroyed by God in the Old Testament, Sodom and Gomorrah.[2]

Sodomy in these ancient writings refers to many, many different things and by no means simply "homosexuality." Masturbation, penile-oral contact, and anal intercourse between heterosexual partners were lumped together with sex with animals as acts of sodomy. So was coitus interruptus (withdrawing the penis before orgasm during heterosexual intercourse, a primitive birth control method), which was also nonprocreative sexual pleasure. According to some medieval writers, heterosexual intercourse in other than the male-superior position was an act of sodomy because the chances of conception were thought to be lessened. Thomas Aquinas, perhaps the most influential scholarly theologian of the Middle Ages, provided the theological underpinnings for these attitudes in his monumental *Summa theologica* and other works, writing that use of the sexual organs for any purpose other than procreation was lustful and sinful. Since homosexual acts could not result in procreation and therefore had pleasure as their only purpose, Aquinas argued that same-sex intimacy was selfish and pleasure-seeking and therefore sinful.

Not all medieval theologians relied on the litmus test of procreative potential to classify sexual sins, however. Many regarded sex between Christians and Jews or between Christians and Muslims as sodomy— even potentially procreative sexual acts could be forbidden if improper partners were involved. This argument derived from the belief that these "infidels" were equivalent to dogs and other animals in the eyes of God; intercourse with them was thus "unnatural."

Medieval sexual categories were different from ours in that sexual *actors* were not classified; sexual *acts* were. A sodomite was not so much a particular type of person as a person who committed a particular type of sin—"unnatural" sex. If the Greeks thought of same-sex intimacy as a pleasure all men and women were likely to enjoy at one time or another, medieval Europeans feared sodomy as a sin anyone might be tempted to commit.

Because the majority of literate persons during this time were priests and monks (an exclusively male domain), and since the church was at times obsessed with preventing "unnatural" acts and punishing "sodomites," only a sketchy historical record exists of same-sex eroticism during the Middle Ages. Nevertheless, there are enough clearly homoerotic letters and poems (ironically, largely by clerics) to suggest to some that a homosexual subculture existed briefly within the monasteries of tenth- and eleventh-century Europe—even leading one historian to refer to "Gay Literature of the High Middle Ages."[3] In later, more repressive centuries, transcripts of "sodomy" trials, and, of course, examination of the numbers of men and women executed for homosexual acts, indicate that homosexuality continued to exist. But almost nothing is known of the inner psychological experiences of persons attracted to their own gender during this period. What, if anything, these persons have in common with modern gays and lesbians is very difficult to say with any confidence.

In various places and at various times during the Middle Ages, same-sex intimacy was frowned on but not severely punished, and affection between persons of the same gender was permitted. At least one of these flowerings of tolerance was sponsored by a particular "bachelor knight" who may have had a personal interest in the matter. The "Constitutions of Melfi," a legal code developed for the administration of the conquered kingdom of Sicily by the German empire in 1231, calls for the punishment of many of the usual medieval religious crimes: heresy and usury (lending money at interest)—but it is conspicuously silent on the subject of homosexuality. The fact that German emperor Frederick II was himself accused by the pope of "sodomy" and of homosexual affairs by contemporary writers has been cited to explain the "Constitutions'" unusual leniency.[4]

Gradually, the Catholic Church came to have greater and greater influence on all aspects of European life as prelates and bishops under the direction of the popes steadily consolidated their power across the Continent. In the process, many "sins," such as heresy against church doctrine and sodomy, became punishable offenses. By the fourteenth century, monarchs and princes throughout Europe bowed to pressure from the Catholic Church to make "sodomy" criminal. Often, it was a capital crime. Thirteenth-century English law called for persons who had intercourse with Jews, children, and members of their own gender to be buried alive. (The same code called for arsonists, sorcerers, and heretics to be burned at the stake.)[5] A church bureaucracy developed which culminated in the establishment by the popes of the office of the Inquisition, charged with the elimination of all those who resisted church authority (variously labeled heretics, witches, or sodomites—as well as, of course, the Jews). Records of the trials of individuals for these offenses during these times indicate that even the most terrifying punishments did not prevent same-sex intimacy from being irresistible to some people.

Historians have traced a gradual shift in attitudes toward homosexuality from the fall of Rome through the beginning of the Renaissance (from A.D. 500 through 1500), from relative indifference toward homosexual behaviors in men and women to gruesome punishments for single acts of same-sex intimacy. The contrasting fortunes and fates of two medieval English monarchs indicate how dramatically attitudes toward same-sex intimacy changed from the early to the late Middle Ages.

Richard the Lionhearted (Richard I), the warrior-crusader king of

England from 1189 to 1199, developed a passionate attachment as a young man to Philip, the young king of France. Chronicler Roger of Hovedon recorded it this way: "Richard, duke of Aquitane, son of the king of England, remained with Philip, the king of France, who so honored him for so long that they ate every day at the same table and from the same dish, and at night their beds did not separate them. And the king of France loved him as his own soul; and they loved each other so much that the king of England was absolutely astonished at the passionate love between them and marveled at it."[6]

Although Richard married, he fathered no children and spent most of his adult life hundreds or even thousands of miles away from his wife. Richard and Philip, on the other hand, spent years together on the Third Crusade to Palestine. Separated from Philip at its conclusion, Richard returned home to England and his family but stayed only a few months before leaving once again for France. He spent the rest of his life there—fighting and ultimately dying in battle against the forces of his former lover. Richard's sexual life did not seem to have generated undue interest during his lifetime, nor did it in any way tarnish his reputation as the embodiment of the valiant and chivalrous knight.

The unfortunate life and gruesome death of Edward II, who ruled over England from 1307 to 1327, could not have been more different. Although he married and fathered four children by Isabella of Spain, Edward's true love was Piers Gaveston, a man often discreetly referred to in older history books as Edward's "favorite." Edward's father, Edward I, exiled Gaveston as an adolescent in an attempt to stop the relationship, but upon ascending the throne himself in 1307 at age twenty-three, Edward recalled his lover to England. Parliament, angered by Gaveston's influence over Edward, exiled Gaveston again almost immediately (1308), but Edward arranged for another return two years later. Rebellious barons eventually effected a more permanent solution to the problem of Gaveston's unseemly relationship with the king by murdering Gaveston in 1312. After Gaveston's death, Edward turned to Hugh le Despenser, a boyhood friend, to whom he remained loyal for the rest of his life. In 1326, Isabella—who was by this time separated from her husband and living with a lover of her own in France—returned to England to rally another baronial rebellion, which this time toppled Edward from the throne for good. Hugh le Despenser was beheaded after his genitals were cut off and publicly burned. Edward languished in Berkeley Castle for nine months before, on Isabella's orders, he was killed by having a red-hot iron inserted into his anus.

Some have argued that Edward was immoderate in bestowing favors on and delegating power to his lovers and that it was his contempt for the barons and his abandonment of his wife—not simply the gender of his sexual partners—which led to his downfall. (Edward was one of several English monarchs deposed and killed by power-hungry barons who used any number of excuses to justify their actions. Another inconvenient English monarch, Edward's namesake Edward V, simply vanished in 1483, one of the "two little princes" who disappeared in the Tower of London under mysterious circumstances.)

As for Isabella, it would perhaps be easier to comprehend her grotesque revenge as the righteous indignation of a wronged wife if she had left her lover behind in France when she returned to take up the barons' banner against her husband. Roger Mortimer accompanied Isabella in the march against Edward and ruled England with her until they were in turn ousted from power by Edward's son, Edward IV. Whatever the politics behind Edward's removal from the throne, the gratuitous torture and mutilation of Edward and le Despenser unmistakably and vividly illustrate the hysterical dread of "sodomy" which would soon sweep across the Continent during the Inquisition and consign thousands of homosexuals to torture and death.

Although modern societies have discarded most of the other medieval rules governing sexual life, attitudes toward homosexuality which developed during the late Middle Ages persist. These attitudes—which originated in a small group of Greek philosophers hundreds of years before the birth of Jesus, were rediscovered and developed by early church theologians, promulgated by the church hierarchy, and enforced by the Inquisition—continue to influence modern attitudes toward homosexuality to a very large degree. Christians are not burned at the stake for having intercourse with Jews or Muslims, heterosexual intercourse in other than the "missionary position" is not considered a sin, and neither is heterosexual oral-genital contact (although it is still a criminal offense in several states). Birth control, which Augustine and Aquinas would certainly have considered "unnatural" and sinful, is forbidden among the main Christian denominations only by the Catholic Church—and many Catholics disagree with this position in principle and in practice.

Nevertheless, attitudes about homosexuality based on theology originating in the Dark Ages persist in our society—while just as seriously held and gruesomely enforced proscriptions against other forms of "sodomy" have been abandoned. How can this inconsistency be explained? The political and psychological dynamics of majority attitudes toward a minority group would seem to account for this inconsistency in a much more compelling way than theological principles. Unpopular rules get changed when they are unpopular with the majority, and unlike the rules against heterosexual "sodomy," the rules against homosexuality affect only a minority of individuals. In Part Four, "Sexual Politics," we will explore these dynamics in detail.

Urnings

As the absolute authority of the church waned during the Renaissance, prohibition against many forms of "sodomy" (sex with Jews, for example) was abandoned. Throughout most of Europe, however, same-sex contact continued to be punished, if not with death sentences, with prison terms and other dire punishments typical of the time: the pillory, exile to the West Indies, even castration. Almost all of our knowledge about the lives of persons whom we might call homosexual living prior to the mid-nineteenth century is derived from accounts of these criminal prosecutions. Several other sources of information began to appear about 150 years ago.

Beginning in the 1840s, physicians interested in mental illness recorded in medical journals descriptions of persons who were persistently attracted sexually to persons of the same sex. (We will explore these writings and attitudes and the development of these theories a little later.) The mid-nineteenth century also saw the first appearance of persons calling for the acceptance of homosexuality in society and for the repeal of laws punishing "crimes against nature." The most outspoken and prolific of those speaking out in this way was Karl Heinrich Ulrichs (1825–95).

One of the first individuals to use the modern concept of sexual orientation, Ulrichs coined a whole vocabulary to describe homosexual persons (several years before a fellow German introduced the word *homosexual* in a pamphlet). Considered in their historical context, Ulrichs' ideas can only be described as revolutionary. Inspired by his conviction that sexual orientation was inborn, unchangeable, and therefore "natural," this remarkably insightful and courageous man tirelessly and unceasingly struggled to change antihomosexual attitudes in Germany and Europe. Through his thoughtful and thorough examination of his own sexual attraction for other men, Ulrichs gradually became convinced that sexual orientation was a stable, inherent human characteristic and homosexuality a valid and natural form of human sexual expression. His life became a crusade to convince others of these ideas.

In reading Ulrichs' letters, diary, and pamphlets, it becomes strikingly clear that the process that led him to his revolutionary ideas was his own development of a homosexual identity—a process that was exactly the same for this mid-nineteenth-century German as that described by modern homosexual persons. He recalled feeling different as a child from other boys his own age. He developed an intense friendship and attraction for another boy when he was ten years old. As an adolescent, he noticed that male nudes from an art book excited and attracted him. Before he was twenty, he recognized unmistakably sexual longings for attractive men. In one of his books, he recalled attending a ball at which there were several "well developed and beautifully uniformed forestry students." "After the ball, when I went to bed in my room . . . alone and unseen by anyone, I suffered real torture, gripped by the memory of these beautiful young men." When he shared some of these feelings with his sister, she reacted sternly, instructing him to ask God to rid him of these unnatural feelings. She pointed out to him in a letter that he had previously spoken of his fondness for one of her female friends. With remarkable and quite poetic clarity, he explained to her the difference between his feelings for men and for women: "The attraction which I felt for her . . . was only a weak reflection of the radiant sunshine of a love, just as the mountaintop gleaming in the rays of the setting sun are not the sun itself but only its reflection." The "sun itself," of course, was the more intense, erotic feelings Ulrichs felt for men.[7]

Ulrichs lived and wrote during a time when sexual contact between persons of the same sex was looked on with horror as a "crime against nature." His revolutionary new idea, drawn from his own experiences, was that love between persons of the same sex was natural for some individuals—and therefore not a crime (nor a sin for that matter): "There is no such thing as an unnatural love. Where true love is, there nature is also."

At his own expense and under the pseudonym "Numa Numantius," Ulrichs published a series of monographs between 1864 and 1869 titled Researches on the Riddle of Love between Men.[8] Each booklet was given a classical-sounding Latin or latinized title like *Vindex* (Victory) or *Ara spei* (Altar to Hope), and in addition to laying out his theories, they contained biographical and autobiographical material, philosophical and political discussions, even poetry.

Convinced that his own sexual attraction for men came from within himself and was natural for him, Ulrichs investigated the details of the formation of sexual organs in the embryo. Learning that male and female sex organs both developed from the same tissues in the sexually unformed embryo, Ulrichs postulated that the "spirit" must also be initially unformed and capable of becoming "male" or "female" in everyone. Ulrichs believed that it was therefore possible for there to be *"anima muliebris virili corpore inclusa"*—a female soul in a male body. He concluded that such a person represented a "third sex." Since no vocabulary existed for this concept, Ulrichs invented one, taking as the basis for his new words a passage from, appropriately enough, Plato's *Symposium*:

> If there were only one Aphrodite, there would be only one love; but as there are two goddesses, there must be two loves. . . . The elder one, having no mother, who is called the heavenly Aphrodite—she is the daughter of *Uranus*; the younger, who is the daughter of Zeus and *Dione*—her we call the common. . . .
>
> The love of the offspring of the common Aphrodite . . . is apt to be of women. . . . But the offspring of the heavenly Aphrodite [Uranian, in other translations] is derived from a mother in whose birth the female has no part. . . . Those who are inspired by this love turn to the male.[9]

Ulrichs coined the words *Uranier* and *Dionäer* for "man-loving" and for "ordinary men" respectively. He later simplified these terms to *Urning* and *Dioning* to designate what we would now call homosexual and heterosexual men. In later additions to his "Researches," Ulrichs elaborated and expanded his theory, eventually developing a complete classification of possible sexual orientations. Women who were sexually attracted to women were *Urningin*. The *Urano-dioning* felt love for men and women, a person we would call bisexual. Ulrichs even coined a term for a Dioning who, because of a lack of female partners, temporarily practiced *Uranismus* (homosexuality): a *Uraniaster*. The

Forschungen

über das Räthsel

der

mannmännlichen Liebe.

„Vincula frango."

Von

Numa Numantius.

———

A title page from one of Ulrichs' *Researches on the Riddle of Man-manly Love*, which were published under the pseudonym "Numa Numantius." (Courtesy of Michael A. Lombardi-Nash, Paul J. Nash, and Eckhard Prinz) homosexual who married because of societal pressures and lived as a heterosexual he called a *Virilisirt*—a virilized (masculinized) Urning. Ulrichs later subdivided Urnings into two subtypes: *Mannling* (manlike), a masculine homosexual, and *Weibling*, an effeminate homosexual; but he acknowledged that between them could be found "thousands of degrees."

Ulrichs was not an academician but rather an activist who had became passionately convinced of the soundness of his ideas based on his own personal experiences and the collected experiences of other Urnings who read his pamphlets and wrote of themselves to him. Ulrichs shared his writings with physicians who were producing medical works on the subject of sexuality and filed briefs and petitions in criminal cases against Urnings. (Ulrichs' reliance on personal experience for his ideas explains to some extent the relative neglect of women's experiences and lesbianism in his works. Perhaps another underlying reason was his society's lack of interest in women's experiences, including the experience of sexuality. Sigmund Freud showed a similar blind spot in much of his own work.)

At the time Ulrichs was writing, in the 1860s, the several kingdoms and autonomous regions that would eventually become united as the German empire had differing sets of laws concerning "crimes against nature." Although the northern kingdom of Prussia had strictly and specifically outlawed sexual contact between men, most of the rest of the German states had not. Eventually, through a series of annexations, treaties, and invasions, the various German states gradually became consolidated into one country. (Ulrichs was imprisoned for several months for his support of the deposed king of his native kingdom of Hanover.) Because of this series of political reorganizations, there were several opportunities to dispose of laws against homosexuality as new codes were developed for new sovereignties. Ulrichs attended the Congress of German Jurists, which was meeting in Munich in 1867 to discuss changes in legal codes, and he was permitted to address the assembly, an event that marked perhaps the closest Ulrichs ever came to effecting real change in the German penal codes punishing homosexuality. By the time Ulrichs spoke to the German jurists, Bavaria was one of the last German states that did not punish homosexuality.[10]

Ulrichs had barely gotten through an introduction to his proposal to the congress to repeal antihomosexual ordinances before cries of "Stop!" interrupted him. He made several attempts to continue his speech, repeatedly interrupted by catcalls and heckling, but was finally forced from the podium by the shouting of the delegates. Delegates demanded that Ulrichs' proposal be suppressed—unread and unheard by the assembly—"in the interest of morality," and the matter was finished.[11] The fiasco marked the end of Ulrichs' attempts at legal reform.

He fared no better in his attempts to influence the medical establishment. Ulrichs corresponded extensively with physicians who were writing on matters of sexuality, including the great pathologist Rudolf Virchow and psychiatrists Karl Wesphal and Richard von Krafft-Ebing. Ulrichs' attempts to interest Krafft-Ebing in homosexuality were quite successful; in fact, Krafft-Ebing wrote a letter to Ulrichs stating, "It was the knowledge of your writings alone that interested me in this highly important field."[12]

Krafft-Ebing's enormously influential book on "sexual deviations," *Psychopathia Sexualis* (discussed in the next chapter), would appear in 1886. Vehemently rejecting Ulrichs' idea that homosexuality was in any way "natural," however, Krafft-Ebing maintained through all twelve editions of *Psychopathia Sexualis* that homosexuality was a degenerate and pathological condition. He regarded Ulrichs and other Urning writers as frauds who sought "to enrich medical knowledge by fatuous gossip about their disease."[13]

In 1880, at the age of fifty-five, Ulrichs left Germany for Italy, eventually settling in the mountain town of Aquila. He gave up all writing on "Uranismus" and devoted himself to writing whimsical stories and pastoral poetry and to editing a newsletter written entirely in Latin called *Alaudae* (The Larks). He corresponded with and was visited by those of the next generation who would take up the now sputtering torch of emancipation for homosexuals: John Addington Symonds and Magnus Hirschfeld. But Ulrichs' ideas had been too revolutionary for his own time, and he died in poverty and obscurity at age seventy, in 1895. By then the German empire had become a reality, and despite the protests of Ulrichs and others, the harsh penalties for homosexuality which had originated in Prussia had been incorporated into the body of law which governed German-speaking peoples from the North Sea to the Alps as "Paragraph 175" of the penal code.

Although Ulrichs' pseudoclassical vocabulary did not come to be accepted, his idea of a homosexual identity did. His concept of the Urning, the "natural" homosexual, contrasted with the notion put forth by others that same-sex attraction was a symptom of physical or mental degeneration or disease. Unfortunately, this view, homosexuality as mental illness, would come to dominate psychiatry—largely through the writings of a professor of psychiatry in Vienna. (No, not Sigmund Freud—we'll meet him a bit later.) A distinguished Englishman of letters and another young physician would offer a different view. We will meet each of these three men in the next chapter.

THREE

Perversion and Inversion

German physicians were beginning to publish reports on and theories about homosexuality by the end of the nineteenth century. By the turn of the century, quite a few "studies" had appeared in scientific publications which detailed the lives of persons who were sexually attracted to persons of their own gender. Unfortunately, Karl Ulrichs' pleas for understanding and objectivity had for the most part fallen on deaf ears. The first scientific works published by members of the medical establishment rejected any concept of "normal homosexuality."

In 1870, a case history of a lesbian appeared in the *Archive für Psychiatrie*, the preeminent professional journal of German psychiatry, which was written by the journal's editor, the German psychiatrist Karl Westphal. Westphal coined the tongue-twisting term *contrary sexual feeling (konträre Sexualempfindung)* to label the phenomenon. In 1891, an entire volume on the subject (*Die konträre Sexualempfindung*) was published by another German psychiatrist, Albert Moll, a work that contains numerous case studies of homosexuals. The source of information on these "cases" was frequently not the physician's consulting room, however—as one reviewer noted, "Dr. Moll . . . has not only been able to fall back on his own medical practice, but has received great assistance from the Berlin police, who have furnished him with much material of great interest."[1] Moll provided information about many of his cases to his colleague Richard von Krafft-Ebing for later editions of his monumental treatise on sex, *Psychopathia Sexualis*.

Not long after they came into existence in the mid-nineteenth century, the new fields of behavioral science turned their attention to sexual behavior. Their conclusions, correct and incorrect, formed the foundations of sexual theory for nearly eighty years—and some of them provided the "scientific" basis for punishing and persecuting homosexuals for just as long.

Krafft-Ebing: *Psychopathia Sexualis*, 1886

It would be difficult to overemphasize the impact of *Psychopathia Sexualis* on the emerging field of the study of sexual matters. A case can be easily made that it was largely due to this book that the scientific consideration of homosexuality remained inextricably intertwined with the study of mental illness for the next eighty years. Krafft-Ebing published new editions of *Psychopathia* almost annually: in the seventeen years between the appearance of the first edition in 1886 and the author's death in 1903, twelve editions appeared. The success of this work catapulted this practically unknown German neurologist into the position of professor of psychiatry and director of the psychiatric clinic of the University of Vienna. Its immense influence and authority marked another milestone in the history of sexuality in Western society: the church had found its position as the supreme arbitrator of sexual normality usurped by a new institution—psychiatry.

Psychopathia Sexualis is a compendium of more than two hundred case histories of individuals who illustrated "the various psychopathological manifestations of sexual life"; indeed, most of the cases are bizarre and quite pathological. Cases 17 through 21 document a series of lust murderers in revolting detail. (Case 17 is "Jack the Ripper," who had terrorized London only the year before the publication of the first edition.) Every conceivable and many almost inconceivable fetishistic practices are recorded, shoe and foot fetishism and passions for kid gloves, lace handkerchiefs, and velvet dresses, among others. ("Fetishism" occurs when an individual's sexual life centers on an object, a situation, such as in exhibitionism, or only a part of the body.) Right after "Breast fetishism" and before the chapter describing sexual crimes committed by severely retarded individuals are about one hundred pages devoted to "antipathic sexual instinct" (Krafft-Ebing rejected the *Urning* terminology of Ulrichs). The term *homosexuality*, suggested by an obscure German pamphletist about twenty years before, appears in later editions.

All the individuals described in this section of *Psychopathia* are indeed involved in some sort of sexual activity with persons of the same sex; however, the range of behaviors is quite broad, and it required a broad conceptual category to include them all. The contexts and details of Krafft-Ebing's descriptions of homosexuals clearly reveal his desire to emphasize the bizarre and perverse aspects of his subjects' lives. "Mr. Z" tries to divert his homosexual desires by forcing himself to frequent brothels. "P" attempts to suppress his sexual interest in men, marries, and fathers a child. He becomes impotent with his wife and avoids sex altogether for several years—then he is arrested in a public park having sex with a young man. Several cases are individuals whom a modern psychiatrist would clearly recognize as having severe mental illnesses but who also happen to be homosexual or are deluded in some way about their sexuality. The most lengthy case study, stretching to almost thirteen pages, is a bizarre account of a man who gradually becomes convinced that his body is changing from that of a male into that of a female, even to the point of experiencing "menstrual discomfort" every four weeks. Several other subjects have all of the symptoms of schizophrenia, and one seems to be a lesbian who suffered from recurrent psychotic depressions.

Despite Krafft-Ebing's statement that his goal is simply to "record" the varieties of human sexual expression, he does not hesitate to propose a theory of causation for homosexuality. He states that, without exception, "this anomaly of psychosexual feeling may be called, clinically, a functional sign of degeneration." The words *neurasthenia* and *neuropathic* recur again and again throughout Krafft-Ebing's case studies, words that were used at the turn of the century to describe the decrepit state of the nervous system of individuals thought to be constitutionally inferior. The nervous system of these pathetic creatures was expected to collapse inevitably and prematurely at some point in their lives.

"Degeneracy" theory had roots in the late eighteenth century but came into its own in the mid-nineteenth century as an explanation for every human foible from idiocy (mental retardation) to urban crime. The conviction that "degenerate classes" of people were responsible for most criminal activity fueled at least in part England's enthusiasm for transporting convicts to Australia during the mid-nineteenth century. It was hoped that removal of the "degenerates" from society would make crime disappear. Alcoholism, poverty, and even labor unrest were blamed on the degeneration of human stock caused by the corrupting and debilitating effects of urbanization and industrialization. (These ideas formed some of the basis for Nazi "racial theory," which would emerge several decades later.)

The language of degeneracy theory sounds like a drumbeat throughout *Psychopathia Sexualis*:

CASE 148. C. age 28, gentleman of leisure; father neuropathic; mother very nervous . . . C. was neuropathically tainted; slight convulsive tic.

CASE 134. Mr. Z., Patient's father was neuropathic, and suffered with nightmare and night-terrors. Grandfather also neuropathic; father's brother an idiot . . . The patient had three sisters and one brother, the latter being subject to moral insanity.

CASE 143. Z. age 28; father very nervous and irritable; mother hysteropathic. He himself constitutionally nervous, suffered from enuresis [bed-wetting] to his 18th year, and was a frail boy.

CASE 163. Miss O., age 23. Mother constitutionally and heavily hysteropathic. Mother's father insane. Father's family untainted.[2]

"Antipathic sexuality," like alcoholism, insanity, and idiocy, was believed to be an expression of an already constitutionally defective nervous system.

Lest constitutionally robust individuals consider themselves safe from the horrors of neurasthenic dilapidation and the development of perversion, Krafft-Ebing presented several cases of "acquired antipathic sexual instinct." Krafft-Ebing believed that masturbation could cause the development of antipathic sexuality in "tainted" individuals: "Perverse sexuality is developed under the influence of neurasthenia induced by masturbation."[3] In reading about them in *Psychopathia* it is difficult to discern how some of the individuals with "acquired" perversion differed from the "constitutional" homosexuals except that they had some heterosexual experience. One man engaged in sexual play with other boys as a child but as a young adult seduced a servant girl and visited a brothel as a university student.[4] Later he had a sexual liaison with a young man and noted that "the thought of females receded more and more into the background." He describes a passionate attachment for another young man who returns his friendship but not his love. His conflict over "having thus sullied this friendship" with sexual thoughts distresses him immensely. Insisting, "I cannot count myself as belonging to the category of so-called homosexual males," he announces, "I have the firm conviction, or hope, at least, that a strong will, assisted and combined with skillful treatment, could transform me into a man of normal feeling." Perhaps it was because such an obviously upright and motivated young man had started his account by stating that he came "from an untainted family" that Krafft-Ebing considered him to be a case of "acquired" homosexuality. Other cases of "acquired manifestation" seem to be persons with various mental illnesses.

Although the biological basis of the abnormal constitution was unknown to Krafft-Ebing, he was confident that its expression could be detected. He believed that individuals with constitutional antipathic sexuality became sexually active earlier in life and that their sexual feelings were stronger ("the sexual life of individuals thus organized manifests itself . . . abnormally early . . . and with abnormal power"). He also felt that "psychical love" in constitutional homosexuals was similarly "exaggerated and exalted" and that they were prone to neuroses and (of course) "neurasthenia" as well as insanity.[5] Krafft-Ebing thus laid a "scientific" foundation for stereotypes about gay people which were to last almost one hundred years: homosexuals are oversexed but shallow asthenics, incapable of mature relationships, prone to mental illness. He used a total of forty-six cases, derived from police records, mental asylums, and other psychiatrists to illustrate his theory and backed up his conclusions with murky "degeneracy" theory and references to "masturbatic neurasthenia."

It may seem strange that *Psychopathia Sexualis* became so influential. Clearly, it was not the subtlety of Krafft-Ebing's insights nor the forcefulness of his reasoning which made the work so popular—if anything, his analyses were simplistic and based on unoriginal ideas already falling out of favor among the scientific community. Rather, it was the hundreds of lurid, seamy, disgusting but titillating case histories that made the book so popular. Here was the sin "not to be spoken of among Christians" described in every detail—and many other "sins" besides. Disclaimers warned that the book was meant for physicians and judges, and booksellers required documentation of same before selling a copy. In the original German and in most of the early translations, genital acts were described in Latin. Nevertheless, the book was so widely available that in later editions of the work, Krafft-Ebing included letters and autobiographical sketches sent to him by readers in England, Russia, and the United States.

Although the methods of inquiry Krafft-Ebing used in his consideration of homosexuality were different from those of Augustine and Aquinas, his conclusions were the same: only procreative (heterosexual) sexuality was "natural" sexuality. Scientifically unsound as his ideas about homosexuality were, they were nevertheless accepted by expert and lay readers alike because they reinforced popular attitudes toward homosexuals.

Albert Moll's 1891 book on homosexuality, *Die conträre Sexualempfindung*, was in many ways superior to Krafft-Ebing's work. Moll had rejected the ridiculous notion that masturbation could lead to homosexuality and had minimized degeneracy theory and "neuropathic taint" as causative factors. But Moll's thoughtful reasonings and especially his steadfast refusal to draw unwarranted conclusions about "causes" of homosexuality and about any association between homosexuality and other mental disorders made his work less conclusive and thus, it would seem, less compelling and authoritative. Appearing in the penumbra of *Psychopathia Sexualis*, Moll's more accurate work attracted less notice and certainly much less notoriety. *Psychopathia*, for all its shortcomings, would unfortunately become the basis of "scientific" thinking about homosexuality for years to come. Psychiatry had joined religion in condemning homosexuals as outcasts and pariahs. The view that homosexuals were mentally ill became nearly fixed in modern psychiatry—only recently, and still incompletely, dislodged. Countless thousands of homosexual men and women would submit themselves to "treatment" based on scientifically untenable theory and data. Today, practitioners of "reparative therapy" for homosexuality (discussed in Chapter 15) follow in Krafft-Ebing's footsteps and those of another Austrian psychiatrist, Sigmund Freud.

Next we will meet two men, contemporaries of Krafft-Ebing, who did not accept his ideas so unquestioningly.

Ellis and Symonds: *Sexual Inversion*, 1897

The story of the writing and printing of *Sexual Inversion*, the first English-language work on homosexuality of any importance, is an extraordinary one, more than worth setting out in some detail. Henry Havelock Ellis (1859–1939) was an English physician whose series of books, Studies on the Psychology of Sex, would eventually make him one of the foremost authorities on sexuality in the English-speaking world. He was contemplating writing the first volume in the series when he was contacted by one of England's most prominent literary figures with a proposal that they collaborate on a book on "sexual inversion."

John Addington Symonds (1840–93) was one of the most prominent figures of late-nineteenth-century England. His seven-volume *Renaissance in Italy* was his magnum opus, but his abundant and varied output included biographies of the English poets Shelley and Sidney and playwright Ben Jonson as well as of Michelangelo. He wrote collections of essays, poetry, travel sketches, literary criticism, and numerous articles for literary journals and magazines. His translations from the Italian of the poetry of Michelangelo and of the autobiographies of Benvenuto Cellini and Count Carlo Gozzi were definitive in their time.

Symonds' own autobiography, or rather, a series of autobiographical sketches that he never edited into a coherent volume, was not published until 1984. Two years after Symonds' death, his literary executor, H. F. Brown, published a biography of the writer based on these memoirs, but he refused to release Symonds' own autobiographical manuscript to anyone. Brown guarded the contents of the memoirs for the rest of his life, and when he died in 1926, he bequeathed the manuscript to the London Library with instructions that the contents remain sealed and unpublished until fifty years after his death.

In 1949, the Committee of the London Library granted permission to Symonds' daughter, Dame Katherine Furse, to read her father's memoirs, kept in "a green cardboard box, tied with strings, measuring at most 6 inches by 12 inches by 18 inches and labelled 'J. A. Symonds Papers,'"[6] but she evidently revealed nothing about the contents of the box to anyone. In 1954, a library subcommittee recommended that the manuscript be made available to "bona fide scholars" as long as "due safeguards" were kept.[7]

The reason for all this obsessive secrecy is revealed in the first paragraph of a chapter titled "Emotional Development":

> It was my primary object when I began these autobiographical notes to describe as accurately and candidly as I was able a type of character,

which I do not at all believe to be exceptional, but which for various intelligible reasons has never yet been properly analyzed. I wanted to supply material for the ethical psychologist and the student of mental pathology, by portraying a man of no mean talents, of no abnormal depravity, whose life has been perplexed from first to last by passion— natural and instinctive, healthy in his own particular case—but morbid and abominable from the point of view of the society in which he lives— persistent passion for the male sex.[8]

Born of the English "gentle class," Symonds grew up in the exclusive Berkeley Square section in London and spent much of his youth and adolescence in Clifton Hill, his family's rather austere-looking manor house in Bristol. A photo of the drawing room at Clifton Hill House shows a large but crowded high Victorian parlor complete with gas lamps, dark velvet furnishings, and a Chinese palm on the grand piano. Symonds was educated at Harrow and later at Oxford and was schooled from an early age in Latin and Greek classics.

As soon as he left the sheltered environment of family life for public school at Harrow (*public school* being the term for an exclusive, expensive private boarding school for gentry), he experienced a sense of isolation and differentness from other boys:

I felt that my course, though it collided with that of my school fellows, was bound to be different from theirs. . . . I had a perfect horror of cricket, football and raquets and I even disliked fencing. . . . I could not throw a ball or a stone like other boys. And oddly enough, I could not learn to whistle like them. And yet I was by no means effeminate. . . . My dislike for games [had] to do with a dreamy and self-involved temperament.[9]

As a young adolescent, he found himself moved by Greek art and literature, recognizing erotic overtones only in retrospect:

With Mr. Knight I read a large part of *The Iliad*. When we came to the last books, I found a passage which made me weep. It was the description of Hermes, going to meet Priam, disguised as a mortal: "Like a young prince with the first down upon his lip, the time when youth is the most charming." The Greek in me awoke to that simple and yet so splendid vision of young manhood. . . . The phrase had all Greek sculpture in it; and all my dim forbodings of the charm of males were here idealized. . . . Hermes, in his prime and bloom of beauty, unlocked some deeper fountains . . . in my soul.[10]

At Harrow, he was confronted with an almost institutionalized homosexuality among the school's boys when he was only thirteen, but Symonds found the "sports of naked boys in bed together" unappealing. "The animalisms of boyish lust sickened by their brutality, offended my taste by their vulgarity." Despite being surrounded by homosexual activity, Symonds "remained free in fact and in act from this contamination." He developed "crushes" on other boys but did not connect these feeling with "vulgar lust."[11] Bewildered and depressed by his conflicting emotions, Symonds saw his health and schoolwork deteriorate in his later years at Harrow.

At seventeen, while visiting some family friends in London, he had taken along a copy of "Cary's Crib" of Plato's works (a Victorian version of "Cliff Notes") to work on during the vacation. Returning one night from an evening at the theater, he went to bed and began to read.

> It so happened that I stumbled on the *Phaedrus*. I read on and on until I reached the end. Then I began *Symposium*; and the sun was shining on the shrubs outside the ground-floor room in which I slept before I shut the book up....
>
> Harrow vanished into unreality. I had touched solid ground, I had obtained sanction of the love which had been ruling me since childhood. Here was the poetry, the philosophy of my own enthusiasm for male beauty.... I now became aware that the Greek race—the actual historical Greeks of antiquity—treated this love seriously, invested it with moral charm, endowed it with sublimity.
>
> For the first time I saw the possibility of resolving in a practical harmony the discords of my instincts.[12]

Several months later during a visit home he fell madly in love with a boy three years younger than he, a young man in the choir of Bristol Cathedral, but Symonds soon came to realize that the "sanction" he had discovered in Plato for love between men was not to be found in Victorian England:

> I could not marry him; modern society provided no bond of comradeship whereby we might have been united. So my first love flowed to waste.
>
> Only too well I knew, alas! that if I avowed my emotion to my father or my friends, I should meet—not merely with no sympathy or understanding or credence—but that I should arouse horror, pain, aversion.[13]

In 1861, when he was twenty-one, Symonds again fell "violently" in love with a young man named Alfred Brooke. This time Symonds could not mistake his feelings for anything else but erotic passion. The other young man was evidently aroused by Symonds' attentions as well, but Symonds found himself paralyzed from acting on his feelings. Some years later, Symonds wrote of the abortive affair in prose that seems high-flown even for a young Victorian: "I spoke to him reservedly—sent him away without one kiss. . . . I lay awake all night, kissing the bed on which he sat, watering the coverlet with tears, praying and cursing in one breath. . . . I roll on my bed in the night watches. . . . The flesh rises within me and the soul is faint through longing. I thirst for him as the hart panteth after water brooks."[14]

The forces that paralyzed young Symonds were the same ones that had stopped him before from acting on his passion for another youth: "I had been taught that the sort of love I felt for Alfred Brooke was wicked. I had seen that it was rewarded with reprobation by modern society. At the same time I knew it to be constitutional, and felt it to be ineradicable."[15]

Symonds threw himself into his studies to distract himself, but his health began to deteriorate again—a fact he attributed to his sexual frustrations. He sought advice from physicians for headaches and pains in his eyes. One suggested for his constitution "cohabitation with a hired mistress or, what was better, matrimony." Symonds seized on this advice as "the one exit" from his difficulties and was married within the year, at age twenty-four.[16]

"A sense of deep disappointment came over me when I found that the *corps feminin* did not exercise the hoped for magic," he wrote of his wedding night.[17] Over the next several years, Symonds fathered four children but slowly came to the terrible realization that it had been a tragic error—"perhaps the great crime of my life was my marriage," he writes in the memoirs. He did not blame himself entirely, however: "I was urged to marry by my father, by my own earnest desire to overcome abnormal inclinations, by the belief that I should regain my health."[18]

His chronic health problems were diagnosed as tuberculosis (by his father, a physician), and Symonds began to frequent Italy and Switzerland because he felt the climate beneficial to his health. As he approached thirty, Symonds settled into an uneasy life of duplicity—his wife, family, and successfully evolving career as writer and lecturer carefully separated from his socializing with homosexual friends, at least one love affair with a young man, and, rarely, a visit to one of London's male brothels. As his lung disease progressed, he persuaded his wife that they should no longer live together, arguing that it was unethical for persons with chronic disease to procreate (an idea consistent with the "degeneracy" theory still enjoying vogue).

Symonds was neither the first nor the last homosexual man to lead a double life. He was, however, profoundly dissatisfied by this life and was perplexed, angered, even obsessed by his dilemma. He also possessed one of the great intellects of his age and struggled prodigiously to make sense of his predicament by investigation and reasoning. Unknowingly, Symonds was traveling in the footsteps of Ulrichs—another man who could not reconcile his convictions that his feelings of love and passion for men were innate and natural for him with his society's condemnation of homosexuals. Searching for answers, Symonds turned to the source of solace and affirmation he had found as an adolescent: the literature of the ancient Greeks.

Greek philosophy, poetry, and art held an interest for English intellectuals of the Victorian age which amounted almost to worship. At the close of the nineteenth century, Britain would hold sway over the largest empire the world had ever seen, nearly a quarter of the population of the globe. The British viewed themselves as the spiritual descendants and natural heirs of the originators of Western culture—an explanation perhaps for the astonishing arrogance shown by Lord Elgin in dismantling the carved frieze from the Parthenon in Athens and sending it on to the British Museum in crates.

Other Victorian classicists glossed over or ignored references to homosexuality in Plato, Aristophanes, Xenophon, and others, but Symonds began a systematic examination of these references, culminating in an eighty-eight-page essay he titled "A Problem in Greek Ethics." In 1883 he published—privately—ten copies of the pamphlet.

In the first paragraph, he comments on the neglect of the phenomenon by "medical and legal writers on the subject, who do not seem to be aware that here alone in history have we the example of a great and highly developed race not only tolerating homosexual passions, but deeming them of spiritual value and attempting to utilize them for the benefit of society."[19] Symonds emphasizes the intellectual, pedagogical, and athletic elements of *paiderastia*, the Greek name for the relationship between the eromenos and erastes (see Chapter 1), and the aesthetic rather than the erotic ("The Greek lover, if I am right in the idea which I have formed of him, sought less to stimulate desire by the contemplation of sensual charms than to attune his spirit with the spectacle of strength at rest in suavity"), but he also makes note of male prostitution and brothels. He devotes only three pages to a discussion of lesbian eroticism and concludes that "the love of female for female remained undeveloped and unhonored" among the Greeks.

Symonds must have hoped that his scholarly exposition of homosexuality among the exalted Greeks would have been a powerful first strike in an effort to begin to bring about change in attitudes toward homosexuals in Britain. But he hesitated to publish his work publicly, dogged perhaps by the worries that held him back from making love to Alfred Brooke, fear of the consequences—fear of the kind of personal catastrophe which would bring down another literary Englishman a few short years later, when Oscar Wilde was sentenced to two years' hard labor for "gross indecencies" with young men.[20] Only Germany had more stringent laws, but they were less harshly enforced; Italy and France did not outlaw any private sexual behavior between consenting adults. "A Problem in Greek Ethics" was not read outside his circle of trusted friends until years later.

In 1886, *Psychopathia Sexualis* appeared, and Symonds, perhaps with the help of his physician father, obtained a copy. He became familiar with papers by other German physicians, as well as French, Italian, and Russian authors. He was by far the most impressed with the pamphlets by Ulrichs, and in 1891, on a visit to Switzerland, he visited the old man in the Italian Alps, by then living in poverty, eking out a meager living with his "little Latin newspaper."[21]

In 1891, Symonds wrote another pamphlet, "A Problem in Modern Ethics," in which he discussed and analyzed the various theories about homosexuality he had collected. Fifty copies were privately printed and distributed among another select group of individuals, who were instructed to make notes in the margins and return their copies.

As he was preparing "Modern Ethics" for publication, Symonds became convinced that he was ready to bring his work to a wider audience. He also realized that he did not have the right credentials to present his analyses of what was considered a "medical" subject and be taken seriously. In 1890 he entered into correspondence with Havelock Ellis, a man almost twenty years younger than he, a physician who had a strong interest in literary matters and anthropology. Ellis had written several articles for literary magazines and a collection of essays on literary figures called *The New Spirit*. It was Ellis's essay on Walt Whitman which had piqued Symonds' interest. Symonds was intensely interested in Whitman's work, especially the "Calamus" part of *Leaves of Grass* with its homoerotic imagery. Symonds proposed to Ellis a collaborative effort to write a book on "sexual inversion," stating, "I am almost certain that this matter will soon attract a great deal of attention; and that it is a field in which pioneers may do excellent service to humanity." Ellis accepted. After reviewing "A Problem in Greek Ethics" and the material that would appear in "A Problem in Modern Ethics," Ellis drew up an outline of the book, assigning chapters to each of them. The plans for the book had been agreed upon and each had just started on his respective chapters when Symonds died suddenly of pneumonia in Rome at the age of fifty-three.

Ellis completed the work himself but relegated Symonds' contributions to footnotes and two appendices: "A Problem in Greek Ethics," which appeared in its entirety, and an essay titled "Ulrichs' Views" by Symonds. As he finished the writing of the book, Ellis started to worry about the consequences of publishing a book on homosexuality in England—where Oscar Wilde was still imprisoned for homosexuality, the "condition" for which *Sexual Inversion* would plead tolerance. Ellis contacted the Leipzig publisher who had issued German editions of several of his works, and in 1896 *Sexual Inversion* was published as *Das konträre Geschlechtsgefühl* in Germany—to little notice. Having thus paved the way, Ellis approached his English publisher, but the work was rejected. He succeeded on his second try, and *Sexual Inversion* listing both Ellis and Symonds as authors appeared with the imprint of another publisher, "Wilson and MacMillan," in 1897.

The ink on the pages of the first English-language edition of *Sexual Inversion* was hardly dry when Symonds' literary executor, Horatio Brown, informed Ellis that the Symonds family was demanding that Symonds' name be removed from the title page and all references to him in the book expunged. Brown went so far as to buy up every available copy of the book (although a few escaped his grasp) and destroy them. Another edition was issued later that same year which omitted "A Problem in Greek Ethics," attributed "Ulrichs' Views" to a mysterious author identified only as "Z," and cryptically identified other contributions by Symonds as being from "one of [Ellis's] correspondents."[22] The new version of *Sexual Inversion* was quietly received by the medical circles for whom Ellis had intended it.

As trying as the conflict with the Symonds family had been for Ellis, it had been a private unpleasantness. Another storm was brewing, however, which would soon erupt into an unmitigated scandal. On May 27, 1898, a police detective entered a bookstore in London and paid ten shillings for a copy of *Sexual Inversion*. Four days later the bookseller, a clergyman's son named George Bedborough, was arrested and charged with distributing obscene material. A "Free Press Defense Committee" was organized by a group of radical intellectuals (including the perhaps not so radical George Bernard Shaw) to defend Bedborough, and the newspapers were full of the affair for weeks. After five months of painful apprehension for Ellis, who had not been charged in the matter, Bedborough was tried and convicted of distributing "a lewd, wicked, bawdy, scandalous libel." Although Ellis's attorney (from the same firm that had defended Oscar Wilde) had shielded him from even being required to testify, Ellis was so rattled by the affair that he would not allow revisions of *Sexual Inversion* or any of the subsequent five volumes of Studies in the Psychology of Sex to be published in England again.[23]

What was so extraordinary about this book? One would think that incredible new information, remarkable insights, or unprecedented conclusions should leap from the pages of a volume whose appearance had generated so much commotion. Instead, *Sexual Inversion* turns out to be a scholarly, measured, restrained survey of history and literature, some current sociological observations, case studies, and theoretical discussions. The thirty-one case studies are clinical, rather repetitive biographies—boring fare indeed when compared with the lurid histories of Krafft-Ebing's driven, tortured "perverts."

CASE XXXI—Miss H., Aged 30 . . . Her earliest affection, at the age of 13, was for a schoolfellow, a graceful coquettish girl with long golden hair and blue eyes. Her affection displayed itself in the performing of all sorts of small services for this girl, in constantly thinking about her, and in feeling deliciously grateful for the smallest return. At the age of 14, she had a similar passion for a cousin; she used to look forward with ecstacy to her visits, and especially to the rare occasions when the cousin slept with her. Her excitement was then so great that she could not sleep, but there was no conscious sexual excitement. At the age of 15 or 16 she fell in love with another cousin; her experiences with this girl were full of delicious sensations; if the cousin only touched her neck, a thrill went through her body which she now regards as sexual. Again, at age 17, she had an overwhelming, passionate fascination for a school-fellow, a pretty, commonplace girl, whom she idealized and etherealized to an extravagant extent. . . . On leaving school at the age of 19, she met a girl of about the same age as herself, very womanly, but not much attracted to men. This girl became much attached to her, and sought to gain her love. After some time Miss H. was attracted by this love, partly from the sense of power it gave her, and an intimate relation grew up. . . . Their general behavior with each other was that of lovers, but they endeavored as far as possible to hide this fact from the world. This relationship lasted for several years, and would have continued, had not Miss H.'s friend, from religious and moral scruples, put an end to the physical relationship.

CASE VI.—"My parentage is very sound and healthy. Both my parents (who belong to the professional middle class) have good general health; nor can I trace any marked abnormal or diseased tendency, of mind or body, in any records of the family. . . .

"At the age of eight or nine, and long before distinct sexual feelings declared themselves, I felt a friendly attraction towards my own sex, and this developed after the age of puberty into a passionate sense of love, which, however, never found any expression for itself till I was fully 20 years of age. . . . The passion for my own sex developed itself gradually, utterly uninfluenced from the outside. . . . My own sexual nature was a mystery to me. . . . I thought about my male friends—sometimes boys my own age, sometimes elder boys, and once even a master—during the day and dreamed about them at night, but was too convinced that I was a hopeless monstrosity ever to make any effectual advances. Later on it was much the same, but gradually, though slowly, I came to find that there were others like myself. I made a few special friends, and at last it came to me occasionally to sleep with them and to satisfy my imperious need by mutual embraces. . . . Before this happened, however, I was once or twice on the brink of despair and madness with repressed passion and torment."[24]

The steadiness of the men and women in Ellis's cases, the lack of anything bizarre or even eccentric, is, of course, the fundamental reve-lation of *Sexual Inversion*. In contrast to reading through *Psychopathia*

Sexualis, at times not unlike picking up a rock and finding all sorts of slimy and grotesque creatures slithering and skittering for cover, the "inverts" revealed by reading *Sexual Inversion* are notable for their normality. Ellis himself states in Chapter 3, "These [cases] were all obtained privately; they are not the inmates of prisons or of asylums, and in most cases they have never consulted a physician concerning their . . . instincts. They pass through life as ordinary, sometimes as honored members of society."[25]

This was a radical new message: except for their sexual partners, homosexuals are not terribly different from everybody else. It is intriguing to speculate on the relative contributions of each author to this message. The text is written throughout in the first person of Ellis while Symonds' ghostly voice beckons urgently from the footnotes with references to Michelangelo and Walt Whitman. One cannot help but wonder if Ellis's final version would have emphasized the normality of homosexuals as much as it does if Symonds had not approached Ellis before the young physician had done much research on the subject. In one of the last letters written before his death, Symonds discussed the collaboration in a letter to Edward Carpenter, a homosexual English writer who lived openly with his male partner. He wrote that he and Ellis were in agreement on "fundamental points" in the collaborative writing of the book. "The only difference is that he is too much inclined to stick to the neuropathical theory of explanation. But I am whittling that away to a minimum."[26]

Ellis dispensed with "degeneracy theory" as a theory that could explain homosexuality—in fact, he discounted it as a theory for much of anything, stating that *degeneration* was a term that threatened "to disappear from scientific terminology, to become a mere term for literary and journalistic abuse."[27] Ellis also dismissed Krafft-Ebing's idea that masturbation could lead to homosexuality.[28] He anticipates later researchers in asserting that "the tendency [begins] before puberty . . . usually between 7 and 9."[29] He questions the idea that homosexuality is ever acquired rather than innate and downplays the power of "suggestion." While not totally dismissing the role of experiences in childhood—seeing them as "exciting" homosexuality—he said, "The seed of suggestion can only develop when it falls on a suitable soil." He was perhaps the first to use the word *latent* in discussing homosexuality.[30]

Ellis was aware of the data from the growing field of embryology demonstrating that, like all animals, the human embryo has rudimentary, undifferentiated sex organs such that "at an early stage of development the sexes are indistinguishable." His formulation of the origins of homosexuality is stunning in its prescience of modern theory, believing that developmental factors lead to a "modification of the organism [so] that it becomes more adapted than the normal or average organism to experience sexual attraction to the same sex."[31] This thoroughly modern postulate of innate biological predispositions acted upon by environmental influences and experiences continues today to be a basic concept underlying the theory of a whole range of variable human attributes—from height to sexual orientation to intelligence.

Ellis advocated abolishing criminal statutes punishing homosexuality and was opposed to "treatments" purporting to "cure" it.[32] Ellis opposed attempts to "treat" sexual inversion primarily because he thought "cure" was probably not possible. He discounted claims to the contrary as self-promoting exaggerations and regarded proclamations of "cures" with deep skepticism. Marriages of "cured" homosexuals he regarded as desperate shams born of the temporary turning away of homosexuals from same-sex eroticism in response to authoritarian and charismatic practitioners. "The apparent change does not turn out to be deep, and the invert's position is more unfortunate than his original position, both for himself and for his wife."[33]

Even though Ellis stopped short of calling homosexuality "normal," *Sexual Inversion* had gone a long way in presenting same-sex eroticism in a less pathological light. Throughout Studies in the Psychology of Sex, Ellis would attempt to demystify sexuality at a time when masturbation was still commonly believed to cause insanity and it was feared by some that the increasing use of birth control methods would bring about the downfall of civilization. In some ways, however, Ellis was still a man of his times—and Victoria was still on the throne of the British empire.[34] Homosexual partnership comparable to heterosexual marriage was just too radical for Ellis (even though his friend, writer Edward Carpenter, had lived in just such a partnership for years). Symonds saw "Greek Love" and the "manly love" of Walt Whitman's poetry as examples of healthy homoerotic sexuality to be aspired to, but Ellis preached continence. It is hard to imagine that Symonds would have agreed with Ellis's closing recommendations to inverts for a happy and healthy life: "It is the ideal of chastity, rather than of normal sexuality, which the congenital invert should hold before his eyes. He may not have in him the makings of *l'homme moyen sensuel*, but he may have in him the makings of a saint."[35]

For all its circumspection, *Sexual Inversion* was nevertheless revolutionary—primarily because it did not present a series of "case histories" of diseased individuals but rather a collection of life stories of ordinary people passing through life otherwise unnoticed. Not until Alfred Kinsey surveyed American men fifty years later would another scientist with so few preconceptions seek out and record the sexually ordinary.

Perhaps the only more radical thinker on homosexuality of Ellis's time was Magnus Hirschfeld in Germany, a physician and psychiatrist who founded the Scientific Humanitarian Committee to advance the cause of emancipation of homosexuals in Germany and whose Institute for Sexual Science in Berlin developed into an internationally famous center for the study of all aspects of sexuality (see Chapter 16). Hirschfeld's call for equal treatment under the law for homosexuals was ignored—partly because he was Jewish but largely because of his own self-proclaimed homosexuality.

Ellis became enormously influential in England and the United States in his later years, and his books liberated discussions of sexuality from the silence of the Victorian era. His call for understanding of homosexuality in particular might have been even more influential had not two men come onto the world stage whose ideas would sweep away Ellis's. The ideas of both would prove catastrophic for homosexuals. Both men were born in Austria, one a physician/philosopher and the other a politician. Sigmund Freud would invent psychoanalysis and Adolf Hitler, the pink triangle.

FOUR

Women's Voices

The voices of women can hardly be discerned among the writings that document the events, personages, and experiences of centuries past. Rarest of all, perhaps, are the voices of women whose emotional and sexual lives centered on other women. Since reading and writing were skills almost exclusively practiced by priests and monks during the Middle Ages, almost all of the existing documentation of same-sex relationships from that time describes relationships between men. But even these writings occasionally hint at same-sex eroticism between women. Saint Augustine, in an instructional epistle, reminds nuns that the love between them should be spiritual rather than carnal and also warned them against "shameful playing with each other."[1]

A few documents recording the love of women for other women fortunately do survive. A twelfth-century manuscript discovered in the monastery of Tegersee in Bavaria includes several verse letters from one nun to another, expressing in sensual terms her grief at being parted from her beloved:

> What is my strength that I should bear it.
> That I should have patience in your absence?
> Is my strength the strength of stones,
> That I should await your return?
> I, who grieve ceaselessly day and night

Like someone who has lost a hand or a foot?
Everything pleasant and delightful
Without you seems like mud underfoot.
I shed tears as I used to smile,
And my heart is never glad.
When I recall the kisses you gave me,
And how with tender words you caressed my little breasts
I want to die because I cannot see you.

What more can I say?
Come home sweet love!
Prolong your trip no longer;
Know that I can bear your absence no longer.
Farewell.
Remember me.[2]

The lives and loves of more eminent women were often thoroughly documented by contemporaries, and occasionally evidence exists which makes homosexual orientation of a prominent woman fairly certain.

Like her predecessor Edward II, Queen Anne of England, the last of the Stuart monarchs, also had a "favorite." When Anne was only five years old, she was introduced to Sarah Jennings, the ten-year-old daughter of one of her stepmother's maids of honor. A relationship began which would last nearly fifty years. The bishop of Salisbury would write that Sarah was "so great a favorite with the Princess that she seemed to be the mistress of her whole heart and thoughts."[3]

Although the two were nearly inseparable during adolescence, marriage was an unquestioned societal expectation to which they both accommodated as they reached marrying age. Anne married the rather colorless Prince George of Denmark, and Sarah wed the ambitious military commander John Churchill. Nevertheless, Anne wrote to Lady Sarah, "Nothing but death will ever make me part from you. For if it be possible, I am ever more and more yours."[4] They continued to correspond as "Mrs. Morley" (Anne) and "Mrs. Freeman" (Sarah) despite living apart. Gushing messages from Anne to Sarah, such as "Nothing can ever express how passionately I am yours,"[5] reveal the intensity of her feelings of love for Sarah, undiminished by the fact that both had husbands. (Sarah insisted that her letters to Anne be burned after they had been read, for reasons that will become clear shortly.)

When Anne ascended the throne in 1702, she made Sarah's husband, John Churchill, the first duke of Marlborough and a commander in her army during the War of Spanish Succession against France. After Churchill routed the French at the Battle of Blenheim, Anne gave the Churchills a fifteen-thousand-acre estate in Oxfordshire on which the fabulous Blenheim Palace would be built at government expense.[6] Despite Anne's generosity toward Sarah and her family, the lives of the two women drifted increasingly apart because of political disagreements that arose between their families. Sarah Churchill increasingly dedicated herself to her husband's career and her children's future and spent less and less time at court as Anne's health deteriorated through a series of pregnancies.

Anne turned for comfort to Abigail Hill, Sarah's younger cousin. Years previously, Lady Sarah had helped Hill secure a position as Anne's chambermaid; now she found that her protégée had become her rival. An unpleasant conflict ensued as Lady Sarah used increasingly nasty methods to attempt to force Anne to renounce Hill. Lady Sarah sent the queen copies of the bawdy songs accusing Anne of lesbianism which were circulating in the capital.[7] A series of spiteful confrontations culminated in a public shouting match between Anne and Sarah on the steps of St. Paul's Cathedral in August 1708.

Despite Lady Sarah's increasingly rude treatment, Anne evidently retained a deep affection for her and agreed to meet at Kensington Palace to try to sort out their differences. Lady Sarah showed up with a list of demands and, incredibly, threatened to make Anne's letters to her public if they were not met. Anne dismissed Lady Sarah from the court (she could easily have had her hauled off to the Tower), and the Churchills left England to live abroad, returning three days after Anne's death at age forty-nine in 1714.[8]

Although a lack of explicit documentation of a sexual relationship between Queen Anne and the duchess of Marlborough has allowed some historians (and Sarah's descendant Sir Winston Churchill) to discount one, Anne's letters to Sarah and her passionate devotion to both Sarah and Abigail reveal that intense relationships with women were an important, perhaps dominant, part of her emotional life.

There can be no doubt about the sexual preferences of another British gentlewoman born almost a hundred years after the quarrel that ended the relationship between Queen Anne and Lady Sarah. Anne Lister, born in the English town of Halifax in 1791, was from a family of Yorkshire gentry. By the age of twenty-two she had outlived her four brothers and been chosen to inherit Shibden Hall, the Lister family estate. A conscientious and prolific diarist, Lister wrote more than sixty-six hundred pages of diaries and journals, much in a code she invented herself. The diaries, which had been packed away in the Halifax archives for centuries before being decoded and transcribed by the dedicated English antiquarian Helena Whitbread, are an extraordinary document of the life and romances of a woman who loved other women in early-nineteenth-century Yorkshire.[9]

A vigorous horsewoman, an exuberant hiker, and a crack shot, Lister pursued these countryside pastimes with a robust masculine style that earned her the sobriquet "Gentleman Jack" from the Halifax townspeople.[10] The love of her life was Marianna Belcome, a gentlewoman from Yorkshire's cathedral city of York, who was not quite a year older than Anne. Lister was twenty-one when they met, and within months of their meeting, the two became lovers. For several years, they enjoyed an idyllic relationship, one that came to an abrupt end when Marianna married Charles Lawton, a wealthy landowner from neighboring Chelshire, in 1816. Lister was devastated, confiding in her diary, "The time, the manner of her marriage . . . Oh, how it broke the magic of my faith forever. How, [in] spite of love, it burst the spell that bound my very reason."[11] The two women managed to meet occasionally, and Lister continued to write passionate letters to Marianna. But their relationship would never be the same. The women had some hope that Charles, almost thirty years older than the two, would die soon and that they could combine the assets of their estates and live together.

A letter alluding to this plan was unfortunately discovered by Charles Lawton in the spring of 1817. "At present, we are in constant fear of him forbidding [Marianna] from writing to me at all. God help those who are tied to such people," Lister wrote at the time.[12] She limited herself to two letters a month for a time: "Till [Charles'] jealous fit subsides a bit, till he gives up fetching the letters himself and till we can therefore write in more security."[13] For good measure, she started to encrypt her letters to Marianna in a code she invented for the purpose. With this added safeguard in place, her letters became more passionate than ever: "Mary, you cannot doubt the love of one who has waited for you so long and patiently. You can give me all the happiness I care for and, pressed to the heart which I believe my own, caressed and treasured there, I will indeed be constant, and never from that moment feel a wish or thought for any other than my wife. . . . Mary, there is a nameless tie in that soft intercourse which blends us into one, and makes me feel that you are mine."[14]

Despite her declarations of constancy, Lister was too passionate to remain satisfied for very long with only letters and infrequent meetings with Marianna: "Could not sleep last night. Dozing, hot and disturbed . . . a violent longing for a female companion came over me, never remember feeling it so painfully before. . . . It was absolute pain to me."[15] During a trip to Paris in 1824, Lister met a lesbian named Maria Barlow with whom she would have another intense and tempestuous relationship.

Anne Lister's matter-of-fact acceptance of her unconventional sexual desires is documented by the forthright, almost breezy style of her diaries. The entries describing her sexual exploits leave nothing to the imagination—some are downright bawdy: "I had kissed and pressed [Maria] on my knee until I had a complete fit of passion. My knees and thighs shook, my breathing and everything told her what was the matter. I then leaned on her bosom and, pretending to sleep, kept pottering about and rubbing the surface of her [vulva]. Then made several attempts to put my hand up her petticoats, which, however, she prevented."[16] Absent from Lister's diaries are anything like the agonized self-recriminations about homosexuality which John Addington Symonds set down in his.

In an 1824 entry, Lister set down a discussion about her sexual orientation toward women. She began by mentioning an affair she had with another schoolgirl as an adolescent:

[I] went to the Manor School and became attached to Eliza Raine. Said how [lesbianism] was all nature. Had it not been genuine the [affair] would have been different. [I] said I had thought much, studied anatomy, etc. Could not find it out. Could not understand myself . . . No exterior formation accounted for it. Alluded to there being an internal correspondence or likeness of the male or female organs of generation. Alluded to the [testes] not slipping through the [inguinal] ring till after birth, etc.[17]

Although certainly not the lengthy explication Ulrichs would attempt about fifty years later, these sentences seem to be Lister's attempt to explain her homosexuality as stemming from a variation of sexual development. She thought of her homosexual feelings as the expression of a masculine essence within her, much as Ulrichs would talk of his feelings for men as arising from a "female soul in a male body." She frequently wrote of her "manly" feelings and sometimes even fantasized about having male genitalia with which to make love to women: "Foolish fancying about Caroline Greenwood, meeting her on Skircoat Moor, taking her into a shed that is there and being connected [having sex] with her. Supposing myself in men's clothes and having a penis."[18] Another time, after she receives a passionate letter from another woman she had met in Paris, she wrote, "Thinking of Mrs. Milne. Fancying I had a penis and was intriguing with her in the downstairs water-closet at Langton before breakfast, to which she would have made no objection."[19]

Lister appears never to have communicated anything about her sexual orientation to anyone other than her lovers. Although her diaries reveal that lesbianism was something known and whispered about even among the gentry, this variation of female sexuality was something that Anne and her contemporaries evidently felt needed to be kept well hidden.

In 1840 Anne Lister traveled east through Europe with another wealthy unmarried heiress named Anne Walker. They embarked excitedly on what was to have been a tour of the Orient and imperial Russia—but Lister suddenly fell ill. She died of a plaguelike illness in the foothills of the Caucasus Mountains not quite fifty years old; her diaries left behind document a vibrant life led largely on its own terms.

Three years before Anne Lister's death, Victoria had ascended the British throne, ushering in an era whose name has become synonymous with repression of sexuality. The Victorian view on female sexuality was that the sex drive was predominantly a masculine instinct and that women, except for "wanton" women, did not have much in the way of sexual appetite.

Throughout most of the eighteenth and nineteenth centuries, women, especially middle- and upper-class women, were thought not to be "naturally" sexual but instead, as one historian put it, "loving but without sexual needs, morally pure, disinterested, benevolent and self-sacrificing."[20] These attitudes and beliefs inevitably affected the way many women thought about and expressed their sexual feelings— many suppressed and sublimated their sexuality almost entirely. The Victorian feminine ideal was the "sentimental" woman: loving but pure, emotionally passionate but chaste. Since heterosexual relationships were considered to be contaminated by the carnal desires of men, women were thought to be able to express their sentimental nature more completely in their relationships with their children and with their women friends. These attitudes may have encouraged the expression of lesbian feelings among more homoerotically oriented women, especially since intense emotional bonds between women were not stigmatized or even discouraged.

A long history of romantic friendships can be discerned in the lives and writings of many women through the eighteenth and nineteenth centuries. Literary historian Lillian Faderman compares these usually nonsexual but nonetheless passionate relationships to more modern concepts of female homosexuality in this way:

> It is likely that most love relationships between women during previous eras, when females were encouraged to force any sexual drive they might have to remain latent, were less physical than they are in our times. But the lack of overtly sexual expression in these romantic friendships should not discount the seriousness or the intensity of the women's passions toward each other—or the fact that if by "lesbian" we mean an all-consuming emotional relationship in which two women are devoted to each other above all else, these ubiquitous . . . romantic friendships were "lesbian."[21]

American poet Emily Dickinson's passionate letters to her future sister-in-law Sue Gilbert reveal the intensity of these romantic friendships:

> Susie, will you indeed come home next Saturday, and be my own again, and kiss me as you used to? Shall I indeed behold you, not "darkly, but face to face" or am I fancying so, and dreaming blessed dreams from which the day will wake me? I hope for you so much and feel so eager for you, feel that I cannot wait, feel that now I must have you—that the expectation once more to see your face again, makes me feel hot and feverish, and my heart beats so fast—I go to sleep at night, and the first thing I know, I am sitting there wide awake, and clasping my hands tightly, and thinking of next Saturday.[22]

Love and devotion between women were accepted, even encouraged by men, who, far from being threatened by them, thought love relationships between women refined and pure, innocent and charming— and utterly without sexual overtones.

Sarah Ponsonby and Eleanor Butler had the ideal romantic friendship. Two upper-class Irishwomen, they eloped from their parents' homes in 1778 disguised in men's clothes and eventually settled together in the Welsh countryside. For the next fifty-three years, they were inseparable, living an idyllic existence in a country cottage as "the Ladies of Llangollen," tending their garden and being visited by the likes of William Wordsworth, Sir Walter Scott, Lady Caroline Lamb, and the duke of Wellington.[23] Their friendship was the inspiration of poets and novelists, and for the next hundred years, women wanting to escape to a lovely country cottage with a romantic friend dreamed of running away like the Ladies of Llangollen. One of their visitors was Anne Lister, who in 1822 recorded in her diary suspicions that the bond between the Ladies of Llangollen was more than mere friendship: "I cannot help thinking that surely [the relationship between Ponsonby and Butler] was not platonic. Heaven forgive me, but I look within myself and doubt. I feel the infirmity of our nature and hesitate to pronounce such attachments un-cemented by something more tender still than friendship."[24]

In late-nineteenth-century New England, long-term monogamous relationships between unmarried women were termed "Boston marriages." One such "marriage" was that between social reform activist Jane Addams and American philanthropist Mary Rozet Smith, a relationship that lasted forty years. By this time, women were not content merely to garden. In the 1880s, Addams had founded Hull House, the premier example of the American settlement house social reform movement in Chicago, an effort that would later earn her the Nobel Peace Prize. The wealthy Mary Smith came to Hull House to join the movement in 1890, and by 1893 Mary was Jane's traveling companion on her famous lecture tours. In a 1902 letter to Mary written during a three-week separation, Jane says wistfully, "You must know dear, how I long for you all the time, and especially during the last three weeks. There is reason in the habit of married folks keeping together."[25] Addams and Smith slept in the same bed in their home, and when they traveled together, Addams wired ahead to be sure they would get a hotel room with a double bed.

A similar union joined two young women from wealthy Baltimore families, Martha Carey Thomas and Mary Garrett, during a time when women were even less content to escape the world of men and sought instead to change it. Thomas, unable to enter the Johns Hopkins University to obtain her graduate degree, went to Europe instead and received a Ph.D. from the University of Vonrich, one of the few universities in the world which at the time granted graduate degrees to women. Upon returning to the United States in 1882, Thomas joined the English faculty of Bryn Mawr College and was soon appointed dean. Garrett, heiress to the Baltimore and Ohio Railroad fortune, had fallen in love with Thomas years before, and when Thomas was a candidate for the presidency of Bryn Mawr, Garrett wrote to the trustees offering to donate ten thousand dollars a year to the college: "Whenever Miss M. Carey Thomas should become president of your college . . . so long as I live and she remains president."[26] Thomas indeed became the first woman president of Bryn Mawr, and Garrett shared a campus home with her from 1894 until Garrett's death in 1915. Thomas called Garrett the source of her "greatest happiness" who was responsible for her "ability to do work" and wrote to her, "A word or a photo does all, and the pulses beat and heart longs in the same old way."[27]

In 1890, the Johns Hopkins University was rescued from the brink of financial ruin by another "strings attached" donation from Garrett. When the original bequest by Quaker philanthropist Johns Hopkins proved insufficient to finance the building of the medical school, Thomas and Garrett, both daughters of trustees of the university, organized the Women's Fund Committee to raise the half million dollars needed to break ground—Garrett contributed about three hundred thousand dollars of her own funds.[28] The committee made one stipulation: the medical school had to admit women on equal terms with men. Despite the initial opposition of the president of the university, the contribution and the stipulation were accepted.

Were these emotionally passionate relationships physically passionate as well? The comments of Anne Lister about the Ladies of Llangollen would suggest they were. Can the relationships of Addams and Smith and Thomas and Garrett be called "lesbian" relationships? Quoting Faderman again: "Whether these unions sometimes or often included sex we will never know, but we do know that these women spent their lives primarily with other women, they gave to other women the bulk of their energy and they formed powerful emotional ties with other women. If their personalities could be projected to our times, it is probable that they should see themselves as 'women-identified women,' i.e., what we would call lesbians, regardless of the level of their sexual interests."[29]

Romantic friendships between women were tolerated, even praised, as long as the dominant cultural image of woman was of a nonsexual creature. Novels depicted pairs of women who eschewed the company of men and remained devoted only to each other. Enid, one of the heroines of Florence Converse's 1897 novel *Diana Victrix*, tells a would-be male suitor: "I am not domestic the way some women are. I shouldn't like to keep house and sew. . . . It would bore me. I should hate it! Sylvia and I share the responsibility here, and the maid works faithfully. There are only a few rooms. We have time for our real work, but a wife wouldn't have. And oh, I couldn't be just a wife! I don't want to! Please go away! I have chosen my life and I love it!"[30]

Novels by male authors such as Henry Wadsworth Longfellow and Henry James also depicted such friendships sympathetically. In James's *The Bostonians* (1885), Olivia Chancellor, a wealthy young woman, forms a passionate attachment to Verena, another young woman, and implores her, "Will you be my friend, my friend of friends, beyond everyone, everything, forever and forever?"[31]

Since women were thought to be practically asexual, the idea that women could be sexual without men was simply too fantastic to consider. In 1811, two mistresses of a girls' boarding school in Scotland were cleared of charges of lesbianism at least in part because the judges found the idea of sex between women simply inconceivable.[32] Even behavior that we would unambiguously label same-sex eroticism between women was usually labeled something else. British and American physicians wrote of young women, often schoolgirls or college women, who slept together and stimulated each other sexually—but called these women masturbators, not lesbians.[33] Since university education was practically unheard of for women before the turn of the nineteenth century and female scientists and physicians vanishingly rare, the experiences of lesbians were largely described and discussed by male physicians and psychologists. Because no women scientists were able to get their writings published, there are no scientific works from this era on the subject of female sexuality written by women. Neither were there female counterparts of Karl Ulrichs or John Addington Symonds—no lesbians were able to publish views on same-sex eroticism at their own expense or collaborate with medical writers to produce accurate and more sympathetic descriptions of lesbian experiences and lives.

Consequently, when Karl Westfal's article on lesbianism appeared in a psychiatric journal in 1870, an article that discussed homosexuality as a form of mental illness, society's tolerance of romantic friendships between women started to wane. By the turn of the century, the female "invert" had been identified, and intense friendships between women began to arouse suspicion, especially if one of the women showed signs of "inversion," that is, masculine characteristics. As Richard von Krafft-Ebing wrote in *Psychopathia Sexualis*:

> [Homosexuality] may nearly always be suspected in females wearing their hair short, or who dress in the fashion of men, or pursue the sports and pastimes of their male acquaintances; also in opera singers and actresses who appear in male attire on the stage by preference . . . the female [homosexual] may be chiefly found in the haunt of boys. She is the rival of their play, preferring the rocking horse, playing at soldiers, etc., to dolls and other girlish occupations. The toilet is neglected and rough boyish manners affected. Love for art finds a substitute in the pursuits of the sciences. . . . Perfumes and sweets are disdained. The consciousness of being a woman and thus to be deprived of college life, or to be barred from the military career, produces painful reflections. The masculine soul, heaving in the female bosom, finds pleasure in the pursuit of manly sports and in manifestations of courage and bravado.[34]

Most sexologists (inaccurately) modeled lesbian relationships after a heterosexual paradigm: an "inverted," sexually aggressive masculine partner and a passive but almost asexual feminine partner. The masculine woman was thought quite pathological, but the "feminine" lesbian was often described as pathetic rather than perverse. In *Sexual Inversion*, Havelock Ellis wrote, "These women . . . are not repelled or disgusted by lover-like advances from persons of their own sex. They are not usually attracted to the average man, though to this rule there are many exceptions. Their faces may be plain or ill-made, but not seldom they possess good figures, a point which is apt to carry more weight with the inverted woman than beauty of face. Their sexual impulses are seldom well marked, but they are of strongly affectionate nature."

Before long, romantic friendships between women were being actively discouraged. In a 1914 book called *Ten Sex Talks with Girls*, adolescent females were directed to avoid girls who were "too affectionate and demonstrative in their manner of talking and acting" with them. "When sleeping in the same bed with another girl, old or young, avoid 'snuggling up' close together."[35] Women could no longer ask for double beds in hotel rooms, as Jane Addams and Mary Smith had during their travels together, without raising suspicion as to their sexual normalcy.

The growing feminist movements in England and the United States often attracted women who increasingly identified themselves as lesbians. British feminist Frances Wilder wrote to Edward Carpenter (see Chapter 3) in 1915, "I have recently read with much interest your book entitled *The Intermediate Sex* and it had lately dawned on me that I myself belong to that class."[36] Women identifying themselves as lesbians did not, however, advocate for acceptance of their homosexuality as Ulrichs and Symonds had. Instead, they largely confined their efforts to goals such as achieving female suffrage, obtaining access for women to universities and medical schools, and spearheading social reform movements aimed at improving the lives of the poor, especially poor women and children.

The rise of the early feminist movements was linked in the writings of many men with female homosexuality. Indeed, for some, they were two sides of the same coin. In 1900, William Lee Howard wrote in *Effeminate Men and Masculine Women*, "The female possessed of masculine ideas of independence; the viragent who would sit in the public highways and lift up her pseudo-virile voice, proclaiming her sole right to decide questions of war or religion, or the value of celibacy and the curse of woman's impurity, and that disgusting anti-social being, the female sex pervert, are simply different degrees of the same class—degenerates."[37] Charges of lesbianism were often used to discredit feminist leaders and their institutions. One American physician wrote in 1902 that female boarding schools and colleges were "the great breeding grounds of artificial [acquired] homosexuality."[38] Dr. James Weir, in an article in *American Naturalist*, wrote that every woman who had been "at all prominent in advancing the cause of equal rights" had "given evidence of masculo-femininity, or [had] shown, conclusively, that she was the victim of psycho-sexual aberrancy."[39]

But if they could not be heard as scientists or physicians, or even feminists, lesbians could and did make their voices heard as novelists and poets. The title character of Virginia Woolf's remarkable surrealistic novel *Orlando* is a young man who is reincarnated as a woman and then re-reincarnated as an androgynous female. Blurring the boundaries of time and gender, *Orlando* is an exploration of female sexuality combining feminism, homoeroticism, and romance. American authors Amy Lowell and Gertrude Stein wrote poetry and short stories about lesbian love in the 1910s and 1920s but encrypted the homoeroticism of these works with ambiguous gender references and secret codes. (In several of her poems, Gertrude Stein uses the word *cow* to mean *orgasm*, as in the poem "As a Wife Has a Cow: A Love Story.")[40]

Perhaps the most famous of these early lesbian voices was that of British novelist Radclyffe Hall, whose best-known work is her 1928 novel *The Well of Loneliness*. Hall lived in Paris with her lover, Una, Lady Troubridge, among a circle of women which included the French writer Colette, author of *Gigi*, and the American writer Gertrude Stein and her lover, Alice B. Toklas. Not unlike John Addington Symonds, Hall had already acquired something of a literary reputation before she became bold enough to attempt a work on homosexuality; *Well* would be her fifth novel. Also like Symonds, Hall wrote this book with the clear intention of winning the acceptance of her contemporaries for homosexuality. "I wrote the book from a deep sense of duty. I am proud indeed to have taken up my pen in defense of those who are utterly defenseless, who being from birth a people set apart in accordance with some hidden scheme of Nature, need all the help that society can give them."[41]

The Well of Loneliness's rich and complex collection of characters and meandering plot center about a woman with a traditionally masculine name of Stephen Gordon. As a seven-year-old girl, Stephen develops a passionate admiration for one of her mother's maids. When the maid kisses her on impulse, Stephen is filled with something "vast, that the mind of seven years found no name for." The "something" is, of course, the awakening of her eroticism. References in the book to contemporary sexologists unambiguously clarifies Stephen's feelings before she herself has: Stephen's father reads pamphlets by Karl Ulrichs. Later Stephen herself reads Krafft-Ebing and recognizes herself. Sensual and passionate, *The Well of Loneliness* is nevertheless tame even by 1928 standards. When after several hundred pages Stephen finally goes to bed with another woman, the reader is simply told, "And that night they were not divided."

Hall's sympathetic portrayal of a lesbian got her into trouble with the English courts after the novel became the target of a public denunciation by one of London's most popular newspapers. The book had been published to good reviews and was selling well when the *Sunday Express* published a photograph of Hall in men's clothing, with short hair and a cigarette, with the headline "A Book That Must Be Suppressed." James Douglas, the editor of the *Express*, wrote:

> This pestilence [homosexuality] is devastating the younger generation. It is wrecking young lives. It is defiling young souls.
>
> . . . [*The Well of Loneliness*] is a seductive and insidious piece of special pleading designed to display perverted decadence as a martyrdom inflicted upon these outcasts by a cruel society; it flings a veil of sentiment over their depravity. It even suggests that their self-made abasement is unavoidable, because they cannot save themselves.
>
> . . . If Christianity does not destroy this doctrine, then this doctrine will destroy it, together with the civilization which it has built upon the ruins of paganism.[42]

After being identified in a popular newspaper as a book that might bring down Christianity and Western civilization, *Well* could not be ignored by the authorities, and Hall was in court within sixty days. Her attorney (who eighteen years later would sit as one of the British judges on the Nuremberg Tribunal) tried to argue the book's literary merits but was not allowed to call his lineup of writers and editors because the magistrate ruled that "it does not follow that because a work is a work of art it is not obscene." In the end, the magistrate ruled the novel obscene, not because it was erotic, not even because it was homoerotic, but because it did not condemn homoeroticism: "The mere fact that a book deals with unnatural offenses between women does not make it obscene. It might even have a strong moral influence, but in the present case there is not one word which suggests that anyone with the horrible tendencies described is in the least degree blameworthy. All the characters are presented as attractive people and put forward with admiration."[43]

Radclyffe Hall saw her novel banned in England for thirty-one years because she had dared to state in a work of fiction what Ellis and Symonds had stated as a matter of fact in *Sexual Inversion*: most homosexuals are ordinary people, not depraved monsters. American publisher Alfred A. Knopf had already typeset the book for American publication when the London trial ended in Hall's defeat. Knopf now balked at publishing the book, and the publication rights were picked up by a fledgling American firm called Covici-Friede. One of the partners of Covici-Friede purposely sent a copy of the book to the New York Society for the Prevention of Vice to instigate an American censorship fight in the courts—hoping the notoriety would boost sales. The ploy worked like a charm, and the book was an immediate best-seller. Ultimately, the society lost its case; *The Well of Loneliness* was never banned in the United States. Hall and Lady Troubridge retired after the London trial to the south of France and later to Italy, where Hall wrote another novel.

In one sense, Hall was more successful with her message than Ellis and Symonds were with theirs. Her book was, despite—or perhaps because of—the English ban, more widely available and thus more widely read. (By the time English authorities allowed *Well* to be published in England in 1968, more than half a million copies of the novel had sold in fourteen languages.) Modern feminist writers have some-times criticized *Well* as overly influenced by the sexist and antihomo-sexual attitudes of the sexologists. Hall's portrayal of lesbians as usually unhappy and defective creatures can be seen as apologetic and full of self-loathing. (At one point in the novel, after Stephen Gordon reads Krafft-Ebing, she laments, "And there are so many of us—thousands of miserable unwanted people . . . hideously maimed and ugly—God's cruel, He let us get flawed in the making.")[44] Nevertheless, being the story of a woman's life, her thoughts, emotions, and loves as well as her disappointments, *The Well of Loneliness* provided encouragement and validation to lesbians about their sexuality which political and scien-tific works, however sympathetic, could not.

Passionate friendships between women became unacceptable as soon as women in these relationships appropriated what had pre-viously been thought of as an exclusively masculine prerogative: sexual expression. The Ladies of Llangollen, who were thought to be chastely tending their garden in Wales and writing poems of devotion to each other, did not threaten Victorian sexual roles. Radclyffe Hall, wearing men's clothing and smoking cigarettes, living openly with her lover and writing about women being sexual without men, became a lightning rod for the uneasiness about female sexuality which the writings of the sexologists had unleashed. At the turn of the nineteenth century, another male physician would take up where Krafft-Ebing had left off in accelerating the process of "medicalizing" lesbianism—as well as male homosexuality. He was a young neurologist from Vienna named Sigmund Freud.

FIVE

Psychoanalysis

In fin-de-siècle Vienna, where Emperor Franz Josef still ruled the Hapsburg empire and Johann Strauss still penned waltz tunes that swept the Continent, Sigmund Freud (1856–1939), a physician by training and a philosopher and an art collector by avocation, would invent a new science of behavior: psychoanalysis. Psychoanalytic theory dominated the behavioral sciences for eighty years and laid the theoretical groundwork for the practice of psychotherapy; even today its profoundly insightful and revolutionary approaches to the understanding of human behavior are tremendously influential. Thus, no attempt to understand homosexuality can be complete without exploring the ideas of the father of psychoanalysis, Sigmund Freud.

Freud was first and foremost a physician, concerning himself with the understanding and treatment of disease states. The subjects for his research were patients who came to him for help with their pain and unhappiness; therefore his insights were almost exclusively derived from his work in the consulting room and hospital. Freud was trained as a neurologist, a specialist in the disorders of the nervous system: conditions such as brain tumors, epilepsy, and multiple sclerosis. In 1885, when he was a *Secundarärzte* at the Vienna Hospital (comparable to a physician in training), Freud was granted a fellowship to study with the most famous neurologist in Europe, Jean-Martin Charcot of the Salpêtrière Hospital in Paris. In Paris, after observing Charcot's demonstrations of "hysteria," Freud found his life's work.

Hysteria was the term for an illness that was thought to occur almost exclusively in women, characterized by physical symptoms that seemed to have no discernible physical basis. "Hysterical" symptoms were inexplicable in terms of what was known about the structure of the nervous system. Charcot demonstrated just such "impossible" symptoms at every lecture: choking sensations in a person who could swallow normally, inability to walk in a person with normal reflexes. Some of Charcot's patients exhibited "hysterical fits" in which muscle spasms suddenly twisted their bodies into painful, grotesque contortions—then disappeared as suddenly as they had come.[1] The young Freud was even more astounded by Charcot's demonstrations using hypnosis, during which he could actually make symptoms appear and disappear in "hysterical" patients. There was no theory of the human nervous system which would explain such phenomena.

Nervous impulses were known at this time to originate in the brain and travel through nerves to muscles and glands; the nervous system was thought to operate the body like an animated automaton—beyond that, only mystery. The brain was an unfathomable organ, its inner workings seemingly undiscoverable. The only "cause" of mental illness which could be conceptualized was a damaged, deteriorated, or constitutionally defective nervous system. Imprecise words like *insanity, degeneration*, and *neurasthenia* were used because contemporary knowledge could not provide any more specific or precise explanation. Freud's intellectual quantum leap was to develop a theory of the mind which did not depend on the contemporary knowledge of the brain.

Although in some of his earlier writings Freud stated that his theories of the mind would one day be shown to have a physical basis, he believed that mental phenomena could be understood and explained independently. He spent the rest of his life observing and seeking to explain the various phenomena of mental life.

Initially Freud used hypnosis to explore this uncharted terrain but soon abandoned the technique as impractical. Instead, he asked his subjects simply to talk to him, hour after hour, day after day; they were instructed to say whatever came into their mind—a technique that would come to be called "free association." As his patients described their memories, dreams, fantasies, and fears in a process he likened to excavating a buried city, Freud discovered links between forgotten events in his patients' lives and the problems and symptoms they had come to him to be relieved of. Often the events were sexual traumas: seduction by an older cousin, an episode of impotence, a brutal rebuff by a lover. Freud came to believe that these traumatic memories could disappear into an almost inaccessible part of the mind (which he called the *unconscious*) but haunt the patient nevertheless, rising into consciousness in a symbolic or transformed way. Freud believed that guilt and shame about sexual activities were frequently a crucial element in the development of the symptoms.[2] Symptoms of paralysis might be interpreted as a pathological "solution" to fears of losing control of an illicit sexual desire, or as the expression of a desire to be taken care of by an indifferent spouse. In an unmarried young woman's "hysterical" seizures, the writhing movements might express pent-up sexual desire—mimicking the pelvic thrusts of forbidden sexual intercourse. The interpretations were always based on extensive and intimate knowledge of the patient's past and present circumstances, temperament, strengths, and weaknesses—everything about them painstakingly gathered by hour upon hour of free association analysis.

Freud extended the psychological principles discovered in his work with patients to explain common phenomena in normal people. For example, if a man discovers too late that he has miscalculated and not left ample travel time to be on time for dinner with a sibling he dislikes, Freud might have said that the man's *unconscious* mind had arranged a hostile snub that the *conscious* mind can be quite innocent of, relieving the man of feeling guilty. Freud considered dreams to be rich in material for analysis and reveled in disentangling their meanings from their imagery. A young woman patient told Freud of her dream of putting a candle into a candlestick and discovering that it was broken and would not stand up. Freud, who knew that the patient's husband was impotent, interpreted this dream as a symbolic representation of this aspect of their marital difficulty. In dreams, symbols often represented their opposites: a dream of a spouse's death accompanied by feelings of intense grief might express a (forbidden) desire to see them dead.

Exploring his patients' mental experiences through their free association, interpreting their dreams, and linking their lost memories to present anxieties, Freud came to develop a theory of human behavior which put tremendous emphasis on early childhood events, and he put forth a model for the normal maturational process called psychosexual development. The details of this process and the implications of the model are monumental in their complexity—the *Standard Edition of the Complete Psychological Works* of Freud comprises twenty-four volumes, making a detailed presentation of even the basics far beyond the scope of this brief survey. Nevertheless, some of the main points can be summarized.

Freud believed that infants and young children had diffuse, undifferentiated, but nonetheless powerful sexual feelings and desires, which were gradually shaped and molded into adult sexual behavior during the process of maturation. He invented a name for this sexual hunger: libido, to emphasize that it was a primitive *precursor* to adult sexual feelings. He believed that the normal child, in the course of normal development, experienced a series of maturational crises and that their ability to navigate these troubled waters determined their psychological health as adults.

Freud attributed emotional and behavioral problems in adults to incomplete or pathological resolutions of the developmental crises of childhood. "Neurotic" symptoms were the symbolic expression of unconscious fears and anxieties rooted in childhood emotional crises which had not been properly worked through. Such patients were "fixated" at one of these maturational points, endlessly acting out pathological solutions to infantile conflicts deep within their unconscious.

Freud's treatment for these problems consisted of a laborious, time-consuming expedition into the unconscious via free association called psychoanalysis. (Freud's theory of the mind and the therapy it engendered share their name.) Requiring hour-long sessions four or five days a week for months, even years, the analyst helps the patient confront and work through his or her "resistance" and make connections between the traumas and conflicts and the symptoms she or he came to be relieved of.

Resistance has a very specific meaning in Freud's theory, referring to any behavior that stands in the way of deeper and deeper probing of the unconscious. If the patient is late for an appointment, says he is having a hard time thinking of things to say, can't remember a name—or thinks the analyst is on the wrong track in exploring some particular feeling or event—all are signs that the patient may be resisting the analysis. Nothing is accident or coincidence; everything means something, often in a symbolically transformed way. Feelings may represent their opposite—a fear of something may represent desire for it. Little by little the past is relinquished, submerged traumas rise to the surface to be dealt with maturely and rationally, symptoms begin to disappear.

Freud was aware of Ulrichs' writings on homosexuality and even published in Magnus Hirschfeld's journal on homosexuality (*Jahrbuch für sexuelle Zwischenstufen* [*Yearbook for Sexual Intermediates*]), but he rejected ideas of an "intermediate sex" or "third sex," stating, "Psychoanalytic research very strongly opposes the attempt to separate homosexuals from other persons as a group of a special nature."[3]

Freud never developed a coherent theory of same-sex eroticism—one expert distinguishes four separate theories of homosexuality which appear in Freud's works.[4] The broad outlines of Freud's theories were sketched by Freud himself in his first attempt to address the issue: "Inverts go through in their childhood a phase of very intense but short-lived fixation on . . . [their] mother, and after overcoming it, they identify themselves with the woman and take themselves as the sexual object; that is, proceeding on a narcissistic basis, they look for young men resembling themselves in persons whom they wish to love as their mother loved them. . . . Their obsessive striving for the man proves to be determined by their restless flight from the woman."[5] Like other psychological symptoms, Freud understood homosexuality (for males at least) as arising from an aberrant childhood experience, poor resolution of a sexual conflict, and the relentless playing out of this conflict in adulthood.

Four years later, Freud posed a somewhat different explanation in discussing his treatment of a five-year-old boy who had developed a phobia of horses. In his discussion of the analysis, in which Freud further developed his ideas about "infantile sexuality," he again addressed the issue of male homosexuality:

> It is the high esteem felt by the homosexual (as a young child) for the male organ which decides his fate. In his childhood he chooses women as his sexual object, so long as he assumes that they too possess what in his eyes is an indispensable part of the body (a penis); when he becomes convinced that women have deceived him in this particular, they cease to be acceptable to him as a sexual object. He cannot forgo a penis in anyone who is to attract him to sexual intercourse; and if circumstances are favorable he will fix his libido upon the "woman with a penis," a youth of feminine appearance.[6]

Although differing in some details, these two theories express a similar idea: male homosexuals do not successfully resolve the "Oedipus complex."

Freud proposed that children go through a stage in their psychosexual development characterized by a subconscious sexual desire for the parent of the opposite sex, a desire usually accompanied by hostility to the parent of the same sex. He called it the Oedipus complex, after the legendary king of Thebes who unwittingly kills his father and marries his mother. Freud believed that if unresolved, this complex of conflicted feelings resulted in an inability to form normal sexual relationships in adulthood.

Freud saw connections between homosexual feelings, paranoia, and jealousy as well and published a paper titled "Certain Neurotic Mechanisms in Jealousy, Paranoia, and Homosexuality."[7] At least one of the two patients discussed appears to have had paranoid schizophrenia—a condition now clearly understood to be caused by an abnormal brain physiology, not childhood experiences.

In 1920, Freud published "The Psychogenesis of a Case of Homosexuality in a Woman."[8] "A beautiful and clever girl of eighteen, belonging to a family of good standing, had aroused displeasure and concern in her parents by the devoted adoration with which she pursued a certain 'society lady' who was about ten years older than herself." In fact, the older woman was a lesbian who lived with another woman "and had intimate relations with her." The girl exhibited all the typical behaviors of a young person in love, sending flowers, writing letters, taking every opportunity to see the woman—waiting outside her house or even at a streetcar stop, hoping to catch a glimpse of her beloved. The parents suspected the truth about the situation; in fact, they had already noticed an indifference to young men in their daughter and "were sure that her present attachment to a woman was only a continuation, in a more marked degree, of a feeling she had displayed of recent years for other members of her own sex which had already aroused her father's suspicion and anger." Eventually, the girl's father happened to run into the two women walking together on the street; he silently glared at them but kept walking. Horrified, the girl blurted out the identity of the man to her companion and revealed that he had forbidden this friendship. The older woman "became incensed at this and ordered the girl to leave her then and there, and never again to wait for her or to address her—the affair must now come to an end." The girl burst into tears and ran off down the street. On a desperate impulse she threw herself over a wall and down an embankment to some railway tracks. Narrowly escaping serious injury, the girl nonetheless spent several weeks in bed, and her parents, now terrified at the possibility of more self-destructive behavior, sent her to Herr Doctor Freud to "bring her back to a normal state of mind."

Freud seems to have taken the case rather reluctantly, worried that the girl was coming to treatment only out of deference to her father. In fact, he saw the root of her homosexuality in her relationship with her father and as being awakened by a coincidence—the birth of a younger brother when she was fifteen.

> The explanation is as follows. It was just when the girl was experiencing the revival of her infantile Oedipus complex at puberty that she suffered her great disappointment. She became keenly conscious of the wish to have a child, and a male one; that what she desired was her father's child and an image of him, *her consciousness was not allowed to know* [emphasis added]. And what happened next? It was not she who bore the child, but her unconsciously hated rival, her mother. Furiously resentful and embittered, she turned away from her father and from men altogether. After this first great reverse she forswore her womanhood and sought another goal for her libido.

Freud proposed that the girl's love for an older woman was a playing out of Oedipal conflicts of which she was not conscious—a desire to bear her father's child and a intense hatred of her mother. For this girl, falling in love was not what it seemed. It was a passion born of hatred and incest.

It is probably obvious by now that psychoanalysis employs a unique method of clinical reasoning. Since the patient is thought to be often unreliable in reporting his or her feelings, what the patient reports feeling may be unreliable as well. What a patient says in analysis may really signify its opposite, or it may be a smoke screen of unconscious resistance to lead the analyst away from the path to the "truth." The fact that the patient is being as honest as he can be doesn't help—because only *conscious thoughts* can be reported and the deception may have *unconscious* motivations of which the patient is not aware. The analyst can discover the unconscious motivations by interpreting symbolic meanings. As the analysis proceeds and the resistance lessens, the analyst is able to discuss and verify interpretations with the patient—who becomes more and more aware of unconscious motivations for his or her problematic behaviors.[9]

Freud and his theories became fabulously popular during his lifetime. His acclaim from British and American psychiatrists if anything surpassed that which he received in continental Europe. Though he originally developed psychoanalysis as a means of understanding and treating hysterical symptoms, Freud elaborated it into a theory that could encompass not only hysteria but every mental illness, all neurotic complaints, and eventually every realm of the human experience from artistic genius to politics and religion. Complex and mysterious, literary in style and details, full of illicit passions—incest, patricide, jealousy—Freud's explications had an enormous appeal to all sorts of intellectuals, and as many laypersons as physicians attended his lectures and read his books. Just reviewing some of the titles of his works, *Moses and Monotheism, Civilization and Its Discontents, Totem and Taboo*, one can appreciate Freud's conviction that there was literally no limit to the power of psychoanalytic theory to explain all aspects of human experience. Psychoanalysis was elegant and comprehensive, and practitioners were limited only by their imagination, intuition, and willingness to explore.

As psychoanalysis spread, Freud's observations and ideas about human behavior were frequently distorted and misunderstood. (In 1914, Freud wryly observed that "in North America . . . the depth of understanding of [psycho-]analysis [did] not keep pace with its popularity.")[10] Although Freud regarded much of his thinking and many of his ideas as preliminary and speculative, some of those who took up his methods did not. In Freud's case studies, where he described one possible way of understanding something about behavior in a particular person, some of Freud's students read scientific laws—applicable to all patients (and nonpatients) everywhere.[11]

Freud's descriptions of disturbed homosexuals who came to him for treatment were used by later theorists to bolster their case that homosexuality was, in and of itself, evidence of mental problems. Freud himself did not share this opinion. He articulated this in a letter to an American woman who had written to him about her homosexual son:

> I gather from your letter that your son is a homosexual. I am most impressed by the fact that you do not mention this term yourself in your in-

formation about him. May I question you, why do you avoid it? Homosexuality is assuredly no advantage but it is nothing to be ashamed of, no vice, no degradation, it cannot be classified as an illness; we consider it to be a variation of the sexual function produced by a certain arrest in development. Many highly respectable individuals of ancient and modern times have been homosexuals, several of the greatest men among them. (Plato, Michelangelo, Leonardo da Vinci, etc.) It is a great injustice to persecute homosexuality as a crime and cruelty too. If you do not believe me, read the books of Havelock Ellis.

By asking me if I can help, you mean, I suppose, if I can abolish homosexuality and make normal heterosexuality take its place. The answer is, in a general way, we cannot promise to achieve it. . . .

What analysis can do for your son runs in a different line. If he is unhappy, neurotic, torn by conflicts, inhibited in social life, analysis may bring him harmony, peace of mind, full efficiency, whether he remains homosexual or gets changed.[12]

This often quoted letter did not surface until 1951, when "an anonymous correspondent" forwarded the handwritten copy dated April 9, 1935, to a professional journal that published the letter as a bit of history.

Freud was convinced that it was impossible to "remove" homosexuality and replace it with heterosexuality. In the case study of the young lesbian quoted above, he wrote, "In general, to undertake to convert a fully developed homosexual into a heterosexual does not offer much more prospect of success than the reverse, except that for good practical reasons the latter is never attempted."[13]

Freud's discussions of homosexuality were thus academic musings, of little practical use except as they illuminated "normal" sexuality. In later psychoanalytic writings on homosexuality by other authors, however, Freud's ideas about a few homosexual patients evolved into theories about all homosexuals—patients and nonpatients alike. Later psychoanalytic authors who attempted to elaborate and consolidate Freud's ideas on homosexuality did so without much success, and their ideas fall apart under close scrutiny.[14] Nevertheless, analysts wrote that homosexuals were disturbed in *all* their relationships: obsessive, narcissistic, immature, even paranoid, driven by fear, disappointment, and hatred in both sexual and nonsexual relationships. Psychoanalytic theorists came to define homosexuals as defective in many areas of life—incapable of mature relationships, "fixated" at an infantile moment of disappointment and abandonment and rage, relentlessly acting out subconscious conflicts in futile, narcissistic, shallow, and short-lived relationships. Freud would certainly have disagreed with these ideas. But some psychiatrists used psychoanalytic theory to draw the most sweeping conclusions about homosexuality to justify contemporary attitudes toward homosexuals: like the statement "there are no healthy homosexuals," written in 1956 by Edmund Bergler, perhaps the most prominent psychoanalytic theorist on homosexuality of the 1950s.[15] (In a 1903 letter to the editor of the Viennese newspaper *Die Zeit*, Freud expressed the polar opposite opinion, writing: "Homosexual persons are not sick.")[16] These neo-Freudians were not tempered by the compassion for homosexuals evidenced by Freud in his letter to an American mother, as another quote from Bergler illustrates: "Homosexuals are essentially disagreeable people . . . a mixture of superciliousness, false aggression, and whimpering. . . . [They are] subservient when confronted with a stronger person, merciless when in power, unscrupulous about trampling on a weaker person."[17]

By the mid-twentieth century, Freud's followers had swept aside nearly every other existing theory of psychology, and psychoanalysis had come to dominate the field of psychiatry completely. Other concepts came out of universities and laboratories (Skinner's theories of behaviorism, for example), but treatment was securely in the hands of the Freudians. Just as other details of Freudian theory found their way into the popular culture (unconscious motivations, dream analysis), the concept of the tormented, defective personality of the homosexual also became widespread.[18]

Like Thomas Aquinas had done more than a thousand years before, psychoanalysis came to define and catalogue homosexuality as an evil according to a system based on faith—in this case, faith in the tenets of psychoanalysis. It took two Americans, Evelyn Hooker and Alfred Kinsey, to start a reformation. We'll meet them in Chapter 6.

SIX

Surveys and Inkblots

Alfred Kinsey

Alfred Kinsey (1894–1956) was an American biologist who lived most of his life in a college town bordered by the wheat fields of the American Midwest. He spent his free time raising day lilies and entertaining friends with Sunday evening "musicales" of phonograph recordings. He was not a psychologist or a psychiatrist but a biologist and educator. His doctorate in biology from Harvard was in taxonomy—the study of classification systems of plants and animals. He wrote three highly successful high school biology texts in the twenties and thirties and coauthored a book on edible wild plants. The research focus of his early career at Harvard and then at Indiana University at Bloomington was entomology, the study of insects. Kinsey's research interest during these days was the evolution of the gall wasp, a flylike parasite found in oak trees and rosebushes. For a time he was the world's leading authority on gall wasps (as well as on oak trees). When his career changed and he moved completely into sex research, leaving entomology behind for good, he donated his insect collection to the American Museum of Natural History in New York—it was the largest collection of any kind ever presented to the museum, more than four million specimens gathered from all over the world.

This successful, respected forty-four-year-old college professor had probably never thought about sex research and might not have entered the field at all had he not been asked to design a course on marriage. In 1938, Indiana University asked Kinsey to coordinate a multidisciplinary faculty that would teach a course on marital relationships; faculty members from the departments of sociology, ethics, law, economics, medicine, and, of course, Kinsey from the biology department would each lecture on some aspect of marriage from the viewpoint of their discipline. Because he was such a compassionate teacher and wonderful lecturer, Kinsey's students soon started to seek him out for advice on their sexual problems. Kinsey quickly found that he didn't have all the answers. As any good teacher and scientist would, Kinsey turned to the scientific literature for answers but was appalled at what he found, or rather, what he didn't find.

> As a teacher of biology, [Kinsey] had had his students bring him the usual number of questions about sex. On investigating the biologic, psychologic, psychiatric, and sociological studies to secure the answers to some of these questions as a taxonomist, [Kinsey] was struck with the inadequacy of the samples on which the studies were based, and the apparent unawareness of the investigators that generalizations were not warranted on the basis of such small samples. . . . Stray individuals had been studied here, a few of them there, forty males in the next study, three hundred females in the most detailed of the case history studies. . . .
>
> All of the studies taken together did not begin to provide a sample of such a size and so distributed as a taxonomist would demand in studying a single plant or animal species. . . . The sex studies were on a very different scale from the insect studies where . . . we had had 150,000 individuals available for the study of a single species of gall wasp.
>
> In many of the published studies of sex there were obvious confusions of moral values, philosophic theory, and the scientific fact. In many of the studies, the interest in classifying types of sexual behavior, in developing broad generalizations, and in prescribing social procedures had far outrun the scientific determinations of the objective fact.[1]

With remarkable objectivity, Kinsey questioned the validity of just about everything that had been written on sexual behavior until then because of the very small and often very select groups that had been studied. He discovered that the vast majority of researchers who had attempted to study sexual behavior started out with invalid preconceptions, which resulted in invalid conclusions. Kinsey's students were asking him about premarital sex, masturbation, homosexual feelings, the whole range of human sexual behaviors—for Kinsey, answering their questions with theories and opinions based on the study of "stray individuals" was dishonest and unethical.

Years before the marriage course, Kinsey had been asked to teach a course to high school biology teachers. During preparation for the course he discovered that there wasn't a textbook that he felt was adequate for teaching high school biology. So Kinsey wrote one—the result was a bestseller. Upon discovering that no one had done what he considered an adequate study of human sexuality, Kinsey decided to study the matter himself. As he stated in the introduction to his first book on the subject, he felt that the place to begin was with the study of the sexual lives of ordinary people:

> An increasing number of persons would like to bring an educated intelligence in the consideration of such matters as sexual adjustments in marriage, the sexual guidance of children . . . sex education, sexual activities which are in conflict with the mores, and the problems confronting persons who are interested in the social control of behavior through religion, custom . . . and the forces of the law. Before it is possible to think scientifically on any of these matter, more needs to be known about the actual behavior of people.[2]

As Kinsey saw it, existing work in the area of human sexuality was fatally flawed by researchers' assumptions about what constituted the usual and the normal in sexual behavior. Kinsey was appalled that behaviors like homosexuality and masturbation were defined as "abnormal" and "pathological" without any investigation into what "normal" was like. Kinsey harshly criticized those who made assumptions or drew conclusions before objectively collecting and then dispassionately analyzing data. After the publication of *Sexual Behavior in the Human Male* (1948), Kinsey received a letter from a psychiatrist who was planning a research project on homosexuality. Kinsey responded: "I am shocked and disturbed at the opening sentence in your letter. You indicate that you are 'planning a research project which will attempt to establish homosexuality as a very frequent etiological agent [cause] for schizophrenia.' Scientists do not attempt to prove anything, they attempt to discover what the facts of the universe are, and they accept these facts whether they are in conformance with anyone's preconception or no." As if this withering blast wasn't enough, he added: "I hope you are not going to add to the list of things which I shall have to critically analyze some day."[3]

Kinsey started his study of human sexuality on a very small scale by collecting and writing down the sexual histories of the students who came to him for advice. Since the course was enormously popular, Kinsey soon found that he had collected more sexual histories on individuals than were in any of the studies he had come across in his search for information to teach the course. The biology professor from Indiana, simply by carefully collecting information from his students, was amassing a body of data on sexual behavior which was unprecedented in the American scientific literature on sexuality.

Gradually realizing the importance of his data, Kinsey conceived a grand plan to collect the sexual histories of one hundred thousand persons from different educational, religious, ethnic, and socioeconomic backgrounds and publish a series of studies on sexual behavior in men, in women, in marriage, on legal aspects of sexual behavior, on "the heterosexual-homosexual balance," and on prostitution and other specialized topics of sexuality. Although only the first two volumes were completed and fewer than twenty thousand histories were collected, Kinsey's work expanded by several orders of magnitude the amount of published data on human sexual behavior.

Kinsey's history taking consisted of in-depth interviews with his subjects, which took between ninety minutes and two hours and asked anywhere from 350 to more than 500 questions, depending on the range of experience of the subject. A list entitled "Items Covered on Sex Histories" in the male volume runs over seven pages of small print and ranges from "age of onset of pubic hair growth" to masturbation techniques to frequency of sexual contact with animals. Kinsey and his associates interviewed college students, clergymen, prison inmates, psychiatric patients, YMCA and YWCA members, female and male prostitutes, and church groups, to list only a fraction of the groups of persons.

Kinsey traveled all over the country to get histories and took them from people whenever and wherever he could do so. People he met waiting in train stations, groups to whom he was lecturing, friends and colleagues—all were invited to meet privately in an office or hotel room to give their history. He took pains to interview groups of "special" populations and sought out prisoners and prostitutes. He asked the people he interviewed to introduce him to their friends and through this technique broke into the secretive homosexual community.

A survey is valid only if the group surveyed is truly representative of the group one is interested in studying—a fiendishly difficult thing to prove. Even picking names at random out of the phone book results in the omission of people who don't have phones, thus possibly missing a group of underprivileged individuals who may considerably change the results of a survey. Kinsey's statistics have been criticized because of the uncontrolled method of selecting subjects for study. For example, his visits to prisons and hospitals make his survey less than random, and his results are skewed by the "special populations" he sought out. Perhaps the most serious flaw is that the survey group is overwhelmingly white.

Kinsey recognized these shortcomings but noted it would be unfeasible "to stand on a street corner, tap every tenth person on the shoulder, and command him to contribute a full and frankly honest sex history." (Even this technique would not guarantee a truly random sample of the population as a whole—one might imagine all sorts of different samples depending on the choice of streets and corners.) Kinsey attempted to correct for these problems by having an extremely large sample, by using United States census results to correct his data, and by getting whenever possible "hundred percent samples," a sample of 100 percent of members of a group "not brought together by a common sexual interest," such as members of a college sorority or residents of a rural township or a rooming house. For all their shortcomings, the Kinsey studies were still far superior to the work done previously, and they hold their own against subsequent studies. After almost ten years of collecting histories and analyzing data, the first book was completed—not intended to be definitive but rather a "progress report" of the project. "Now, after a decade of hush-hush, comes a book that is sure to create an explosion and to be bitterly controversial," read the review in the *New York Times* of January 4, 1948.

The publication of *Sexual Behavior in the Human Male* proved to be explosive indeed. Based on marketing research, the publisher had made the monumental blunder of printing only ten thousand copies of the book. Six more printings were ordered in the first weeks of publication, and two hundred thousand copies were sold within two months of its release. Although no booksellers were arrested for distributing obscene literature as had happened with Ellis's *Sexual Inver-*

sion, at least one group, a Catholic organization called the Health League of Canada, petitioned the postmaster of Canada to prohibit distribution through the Canadian Postal Service (the petition was never acted upon). Anthropologist Margaret Mead denounced the book at the annual convention of the Social Hygiene Association, as did Clare Boothe Luce at the National Council of Catholic Women's convention. *Reader's Digest* published an article with the titillating title "Must We Change Our Sex Standards?" in response to Kinsey's book and kept up a steady stream of criticism with a series of condemnatory essays by the likes of Norman Vincent Peale and J. Edgar Hoover (whose personal interest in the subject of homosexuality was still a well-kept secret).

One might imagine that *Sexual Behavior in the Human Male* caused such a furor because it was a compendium of lurid sexual stories in the style of *Psychopathia Sexualis*—nothing could be farther from the truth. Thrill seekers who handed over $6.50 for the 804-page volume published by the staid medical publishing house of W. B. Saunders Company were to be disappointed. The book contained an eighty-eight-page discussion of statistical methods (32 pages discussing the validity issue alone), hundreds of graphs and tables of data, and page after page of prose like "While approximately 3.3 is the mean frequency of total outlet for younger males, no mean nor median, nor any other sort of average, can be significant unless one keeps in mind the range of the individual variation and the distribution of these variants in the population as a whole." So unerotic a book on sex had never been written. Kinsey's biographer and collaborator, Wardell Pomeroy, characterized it as "one of those occasional phenomena in the publishing business: a little-read best seller."[4]

Buried among the thousands of pieces of data were a few statistics that completely dumbfounded the "experts" and most ordinary people as well: 27 to 37 percent of married men admitted to extramarital intercourse, more than 90 percent of men masturbated, 60 percent had had some sort of oral-genital contact. Nothing, however, was as surprising as the data on homosexual contacts: 37 percent of the men surveyed reported at least one homosexual contact to the point of orgasm sometime during their lives; the rate climbed to 50 percent in men who remained unmarried until age thirty-five. Ten percent of males were more or less exclusively homosexual for at least three years between the ages of sixteen and fifty-five. Kinsey wrote:

We ourselves were totally unprepared to find such incidence data when this research was originally undertaken. Over a period of several years we were repeatedly assailed with doubts as to whether we were getting a fair cross section of the total population or whether a selection of cases was biasing the results. It has been our experience, however, that each new group into which we have gone has provided substantially the same data. Whether the histories were taken in large cities, in small towns, or in rural areas, whether they came from one college or another, a church school or a state university or some private institution, whether they came from one part of the country or from another, the incidence data on the homosexual have been more or less the same.[5]

During the years that Kinsey and his associates were gathering their data, it had become apparent that attempting to identify individuals as either "homosexual" or "heterosexual" was simply impossible. There were "heterosexual" persons who had never had homosexual contact and "homosexual" persons who had never had heterosexual contact, but there were many who had had erotic experiences with both sexes. For the purposes of analyzing the data, Kinsey devised a seven-point scale that ranked individuals from 0 to 6 according to the proportion of homosexual and heterosexual activity, including both the physical contact and the "psychological reactions" they had experienced. Individuals rated "0" were "exclusively heterosexual with no homosexual experience"; "1," "predominantly heterosexual with only incidental homosexual experience," and so forth through "6," "exclusively homosexual." Known now as the "Kinsey Scale," it continues to be a basic investigational instrument of modern sex researchers.

Part of *Sexual Behavior in the Human Male* consists of nine chapters that describe "sources of sexual outlet," referring to the means by which orgasm was achieved. Each chapter is devoted to a particular "outlet": masturbation, premarital intercourse, intercourse with prostitutes, and so forth. The "Homosexual Outlet" chapter is forty-nine pages long, nearly three times the length of the next longest chapter (which happens to be "Masturbation") and more than six times the length of the chapter titled "Marital Intercourse." Kinsey apparently believed that the data on homosexuality were the most far-reaching in their ramifications, adding a section titled "Scientific and Social Implications" to this chapter alone among all the other "outlet" chapters. The major implication of the data was that since homosexuality (broadly defined as any homosexual contact) was so common in a nonclinical population, it seemed unlikely that same-sex eroticism was, as had been assumed, pathological: "In view of the data which we now have on the incidence and frequency of the homosexual, and in particular on its co-existence with the heterosexual in the lives of a considerable portion of the male population, it is difficult to maintain the view that psychosexual reactions between individuals of the same sex are rare and therefore abnormal or unnatural, or that they constitute within themselves evidence of neurosis or even psychoses."[6] A broader implication of the data was that "the homosexual" as a type of person did not exist. There were men who had sex only with women, men who had sex only with men, and men who had sex with both men and women. But for Kinsey, homosexuality was something one did, not something one was.

Unfortunately, Kinsey was not immune from occasionally falling into the same sort of error he criticized in others who had written on sexual behavior, namely, proposing mechanisms based on impressions suggested by patterns of his data. In his zeal to destigmatize homosexuality by removing the taint of the "psychopathic" from persons who enjoyed same-sex eroticism, he asserted that the choice of sexual part-

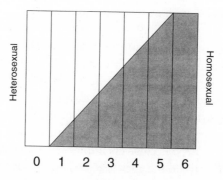

The Kinsey Heterosexual-Homosexual Rating Scale, introduced in Kinsey, Pomeroy, and Martin's *Sexual Behavior in the Human Male.* 0 = exclusively heterosexual; 1 = predominately heterosexual, only incidentally homosexual; 2 = predominately heterosexual, but more than incidentally homosexual; 3 = equally heterosexual and homosexual; 4 = predominately homosexual, but more than incidentally heterosexual; 5 = predominately homosexual, only incidentally heterosexual; 6 = exclusively homosexual. (Reproduced from the original figure by permission of the Kinsey Institute for Research in Sex, Gender, and Reproduction, Inc.)

ners was simply that—a choice, certainly not driven by anything inherent in the individual. He discounted biological factors, especially hereditary factors, in homosexuality and emphasized the role of culture and socialization in the development of patterns of homosexual or heterosexual "outlets."

> One of the factors that materially contributes to the development of exclusively homosexual histories is the ostracism which society imposes upon one who is discovered to have had perhaps no more than a lone experience. The high school boy is likely to be expelled from school and, if it is in a small town, he is almost certain to be driven from the community. His chances for making heterosexual contacts are tremendously reduced after the public disclosure, and he is forced into the company of other homosexual individuals among whom he finally develops an exclusively homosexual pattern for himself.[7]

Kinsey believed that the selection of a sexual partner was largely determined by custom, social constraints, opportunity, and even convenience, an interpretation that was not in any way proven by his data. Kinsey's thinking about the origins of homosexuality would probably place him today among the social scientists who call themselves "constructionists"—those who believe that humans have an unfocused, directionless sex drive that custom, mores, and other societal forces orient in culturally accepted patterns. Such a theory is, of course, consistent with the Kinsey data; but his data certainly do not prove "constructionist" views—neither do they disprove the "essentialist" point of view that homosexuality is an essential attribute of the individual.

Perhaps the most controversial statistic in all of Kinsey's work is the famous "10 percent" figure. Kinsey reported that 10 percent of the males were "more or less exclusively homosexual (i.e., rate 5 or 6) for at least three years between the ages of 16 and 55."[8] This was "one male in ten in the white male population." The problem with this figure is that it is usually taken out of context and construed to mean that 10 percent of the adult male population is "more or less exclusively homosexual." Often, the figure is extended to females as well and the assertion made that 10 percent of the population is gay or lesbian. This is not what the Kinsey data show, and this misuse of the data is a great disservice to his work. Kinsey measured sexual *behaviors*—and did not classify persons as sexual creatures of a particular type. A young man who sexually experiments once or twice with another male adolescent but then becomes exclusively and happily heterosexual as an adult might be classified as a "Kinsey 6" for the several years before he had heterosexual contact. Kinsey would likely have refused to attempt to answer a question like "What percent of men are homosexuals?" because he did not conceptualize homosexuality-heterosexuality as a way to classify persons—only behaviors.

Kinsey's major conclusion about homosexuality was that same-sex eroticism and homosexual behavior did not brand a person as a monster and should be considered neither criminal nor an excuse for ostracizing individuals.

> The judge who is considering the case of the male who has been arrested for homosexual activity should keep in mind that nearly 40 per cent of all other males in the town could be arrested at some time in their lives for similar activity. . . . The court might also keep in mind that the penal or mental institution to which he may send the male has something between 30 and 85 per cent of its inmates engaging in the sort of homosexual activity which may be involved in the individual case before him.[9]

Kinsey pointed out that if the criminal codes against homosexuality were completely enforced against every man who broke "crimes against nature" laws, 6.3 million persons would have needed to be institutionalized immediately. (The U.S. population in 1948 was approximately 150 million.)

In 1953, the second of Kinsey's reports on his survey of human sexual behavior was published: *Sexual Behavior in the Human Female*.[10] Comparable to the data on homosexuality in the *Male* volume, Kinsey's group reported in this book that a large percentage of the women interviewed reported erotic interest in other women. By about age thirty, 25 percent of all females "recognized erotic responses to other females."[11] By age forty, 19 percent of the women interviewed "had some physical contact with other females which was deliberately and consciously . . . intended to be sexual." This figure rose to 24 percent if only unmarried women were counted. By the age of forty-five, 13 percent of women had experienced homosexual contact to the point of orgasm.

In the *Female* volume, Kinsey expanded on and more clearly articulated his ideas about homosexuality, stating, for example, "It should again be pointed out . . . that it is impossible to determine the number of individuals who are 'homosexual' or 'heterosexual.' It is only possible to determine how many persons belong, at any particular time, to each of the classifications on a heterosexual-homosexual scale."[12] He also stated: "It is a characteristic of the human mind that it tries to dichotomize in its classification of phenomena. Things are either so, or they are not so. Sexual behavior is either normal or abnormal, socially acceptable or unacceptable, heterosexual or homosexual; and many persons do not want to believe that there are gradations in these matters from one to the other extreme."[13]

As in the first book, Kinsey included an explanatory chapter on the social significance of homosexuality in *Sexual Behavior in the Human Female*, but this time he used survey data to make his points. For example, he asked his respondents whether they "regretted" their homosexual experience (most did not), whether they "approved" of homosexual behavior in others, and whether they would "keep friends" they discovered to have had homosexual activity (most said they would).

Kinsey stressed the normality of many of the lesbians his researchers interviewed, noting that they included "many assured individuals who were happy and successful in the homosexual adjustments, economically and socially well established in their communities and, in many instances, persons of considerable significance in the social organization."

Kinsey also continued to maintain that the opportunity for and experience of sexual relationships were the most important factors in determining an individual's sexual orientation: "Not a few of the [lesbians interviewed] were professionally trained women who had been preoccupied with their education or other matters in the day when social relations with males and marriage might have been available, and who in subsequent years had found homosexual contacts more readily available than heterosexual contacts. . . . For many of these women, heterosexual relations or marriage would have been difficult while they maintained their professional careers."

The psychiatric community was not so much critical as dismissive of the Kinsey reports. Kinsey's methods and statistical analysis were criticized—often by taking data out of context to make them appear ludicrous. One psychoanalyst gleefully pointed to Kinsey's "conclusion" that 37 percent of men were homosexuals—an utter distortion of the data used to attempt to discredit the entire report. Psychoanalytic practitioners used psychoanalytic reasoning to dismiss data that they felt had been supplied by disturbed homosexuals who "unconsciously" justified their own pathology by unconsciously inflating the incidence of homosexuality during interviews. Psychiatrists asserted that Kinsey did not report on the pathology of his subjects because he didn't know how to find it—that he had not psychoanalyzed his subjects but only asked them what they did sexually.

Almost thirty years later American psychiatry would begin to understand what Kinsey had demonstrated about homosexuality in his work—that homosexual activity was common in many individuals, at least at some point in their lives, and should not be regarded as indicating serious mental disturbance.

More recently, another report on the sexual practices of Americans appeared in print, again derived from survey results.[14] Based on a sample of almost thirty-five hundred people interviewed in 1992, this study found that 7.1 percent of the men interviewed and 3.8 percent of the women reported some type of sexual contact with a same-sex partner since puberty. The percentage of individuals reporting sexual contact with a same-sex partner in the twelve months preceding the interviews drops to 2.7 percent for men and 1.3 percent for women—roughly corresponding to the percentages of individuals who reported that they think of themselves as homosexual or bisexual (2.8 percent of men and 1.4 percent of women).

While Kinsey was defending his work in print and lectures, another American scientist was quietly at work on a landmark study about sexual behavior which would open another chink in the psychoanalytic monolith. Evelyn Hooker used some of the same techniques sometimes used to probe the unconscious, including the Rorschach test—the famous "inkblots"—and would come up with some surprising conclusions, among them: "Homosexuality as a *clinical* entity does not exist."[15]

Evelyn Hooker

In 1958, a short paper in a rather obscure professional journal propelled Evelyn Hooker onto the stage of sexual politics with almost the same velocity that *Sexual Behavior in the Human Male* had propelled Alfred Kinsey there ten years earlier. Hooker's name did not become a household word as Kinsey's had, perhaps because her work, studying homosexual men, did not seem relevant to most Americans. However, the emerging gay and lesbian community, along with a small number of astute behavioral scientists, recognized "The Adjustment of the Male Overt Homosexual," in the *Journal of Projective Techniques*, for the landmark study it was. Hooker's work would be used more than twenty years later to bolster the efforts of those who would eventually have homosexuality removed from the list of mental disorders of the American Psychiatric Association.

Soon after receiving her Ph.D. in psychology, Hooker joined the faculty at the University of California at Los Angeles and taught some courses. Among her students was a gay man she befriended, and in time she was introduced into his circle of friends, mostly other gay men. Hooker soon noticed, much as Havelock Ellis had done years before, that these men did not fit the stereotype of the homosexual: promiscuous, neurotic, shallow, sexually obsessed, frightened of and hostile toward women. This heterosexual female psychologist met and socialized with intelligent, often talented homosexual men—many in long-term relationships—who seemed well adjusted and happy. Her gay friends were acutely aware of what was written about them in the psychology books, and as the relationships between Dr. Hooker and these men grew closer, some of them suggested that she study them as research subjects and disprove the theory that homosexuals were uniformly disturbed individuals. After some hesitation, Hooker agreed to do so; in fact, she applied for and received a grant from the National Institutes of Mental Health to support her work.

Her experimental design was elegantly simple: (1) administer some psychological tests to a group of homosexual men and to a group of heterosexual men, (2) ask a panel of experts to interpret the tests without knowing the sexual orientation of the subjects, and (3) ask the experts to rate the psychological health of the subjects without knowing the sexual orientation of the men they were rating. As an added twist and challenge, Hooker would also ask the experts to determine who was heterosexual and who was homosexual based on the test results alone.

Prevailing psychiatric and psychological theory predicted that the experts would find evidence of psychological disturbance in the test results of homosexual men and that particular patterns of disturbance—hostile or fearful attitudes toward women, evidence of sexual confusion, "castration anxiety," and so forth—would make it easy to spot the homosexual subjects.

An aside on the testing will be useful here. The Rorschach, or inkblot, test is done by presenting a series of cards showing rather meaningless blobs and smudges and asking the person being tested to say what the shapes look like or remind him or her of. The theory behind the test is that when a subject is presented with abstract, meaningless shapes and required to draw meaning out of them, the meanings derived provide insight into how the subject thinks about the world and organizes information. Depressed people will see depressing things in the inkblot: dead bodies, wilted plants; anxious people will see frightening things: bats, snakes, or even monsters; obsessive-compulsive people will describe every tiny detail of the pattern and give many responses. Psychotics will give bizarre responses not even suggested by the card. Several cards have shapes that clearly suggest human figures that are not particularly male or female. How subjects deal with these figures provides insight into their thinking and emotional responses to men and women. The cards are standardized—every psychologist uses pictures of the same inkblots—and the scoring is standardized as well. The number of animal shapes and human shapes reported by the subjects, their overall impressions, responses about details of blots, areas the subjects avoid or can't "see" anything in—each response is categorized and tabulated. When done correctly, the test is quite useful and can accurately pick up many types of psychological problems. "I used the Rorschach because many clinicians believe it to be the best method of assessing total personality structure and, also, because it is one of the test instruments currently used for the diagnosis of homosexuality," Hooker stated in the paper.[16]

Another quite similar test was used as well, the Thematic Apperception Test (TAT for short). This test also involves a series of standardized pictures, this time drawings of a person or persons in various settings. The subject is asked to make up a story describing what is going on in the picture. Again, the pictures are deliberately ambiguous, and the relationships and activities of the persons in the pictures are indeterminate. In making up a story, the subject brings out information about what he or she expects from people and how he or she judges various types of persons, men, women, children, older persons, and so forth.

Hooker recruited thirty gay men from among the members of the Mattachine Society, an early gay rights organization in California. She eliminated anyone who was receiving psychiatric treatment or therapy. For the heterosexual group (the "control" group, or "normals" with which the gay men would be compared), she approached other civic organizations and recruited heterosexual men, again eliminating any men with a history of psychiatric treatment. The heterosexual men were then matched to the homosexual men according to age, education, and IQ. For example, for "Pair One" in the study, Hooker found and tested a forty-four-year-old heterosexual man who was a high school graduate with an IQ of 105, to compare results with those of a forty-two-year-old gay man, also a high school graduate, also with an IQ of 105. Thirty matched pairs of homosexual and heterosexual men were eventually obtained. The average IQs of the two groups of men differ by less than one point—a remarkable accomplishment. One can only imagine how many IQ tests needed to be administered to what number of men to assemble these thirty pairs. Hooker had attempted to match the groups according to their occupations as well but found this to be "manifestly impossible."

Hooker administered and recorded the responses of the subjects and presented the results to three eminent psychologists who were considered experts in the interpretation of these tests. She first presented the results in random order and asked the experts to rate them on a scale of one to five on their "psychological adjustment." A score of "one" meant that the subject had "superior" adjustment, with "superior integration of capacities, both intellectual and emotional, ease and comfort in relation to self and functioning effectively in the social environment"; "three" was average adjustment, "five," "bottom limit of normal or maladjusted, with signs of pathology." The judges were then presented with the results of the paired men and asked to determine which of the pair was the homosexual.

The results were unequivocal. The adjustment ratings for the two groups, heterosexual and homosexual, showed no significant differences. An almost identical number of heterosexuals and homosexuals received the top ratings; if anything, the gay men did better: more gay men received a "one" or a "two" rating than did the heterosexual controls. (The trend is not significant when statistical methods are applied to the data.) Even more remarkable, the judges could correctly identify the gay man in the matched pairs only about 50 percent of the time using the Rorschach results, no better than chance alone would predict—no better than if they had simply flipped a coin.

To drive home the point, Hooker quoted the experts' impressions and interpretations of the testing results in the paper (she had actually recorded them during the interpretation sessions). Here is one judge's interpretation of one subject's Rorschach test:

> [This subject] handles hostility and sexuality easily. . . . He is able to love and to dislike. He is a good husband and father and would be a steady employee. I could see him as having a better-than-average job. . . . He is a middle-of-the-roader. This is as clean a record as I think I have seen. I don't think he has strong dependency needs. He is comfortable, and in that sense he is strong. I imply that this is a heterosexual record specifically.

The subject being rated was a gay man—one who had had exclusively homosexual experiences, a "Kinsey 6." The comments of the same judge interpreting the TAT results for this *same man* provide an interesting insight into the operation of bias in the interpretation of the results: "Here is indecision and a schizoid feeling. There is some aridity. This is not an out-going, warm, decisive person. It is a constricted, somewhat egocentric, somewhat schizoid, perturbed, guilty fellow." This second interpretation is quite different from that of the first. Why? Possibly because the judge didn't know the subject was homosexual from the Rorschach. The TAT, however, requires the subject to make up a story, and it was not too unusual for the gay men to make up a "gay" story—one involving intimacy between men—thus quickly identifying themselves as homosexual. This man had done so, and this knowledge clearly biased the judge when he interpreted the TAT. Although Hooker did not draw any conclusions about this disagreement in the paper, the implication was clear: knowing that an individual is homosexual can be a source of bias for a psychoanalytically trained clinician. He or she often finds evidence of "pathology" where an unbiased clinician finds none.

Hooker drew three conclusions from her study:

1. Homosexuality as a *clinical* [emphasis added] entity does not exist. Its forms are as varied as heterosexuality.
2. Homosexuality may be a deviation in the sexual pattern which is within the normal range psychologically.
3. The role of particular forms of sexual desire and expression in personality and development may be less important than has frequently been assumed.

Unfortunately, very few paid much attention to Hooker. She was a research psychologist rather than a clinician and an unknown one at that. In the introduction to her paper, she had quoted the Group for the Advancement of Psychiatry of the American Psychiatric Association's recent report on homosexuality. This report, issued in 1955, had obviously not been influenced by Kinsey studies and concluded, "When . . . homosexual behavior persists in an adult, it is then a symptom of severe emotional disturbance." The psychiatric establishment could safely ignore one little study by an unknown psychologist from California—and did.

Hooker continued to study the lives of homosexual men and wrote descriptions of the developing gay and lesbian community. She was one of the first behavioral scientists to claim that most of the "maladjustments" seen by clinicians in gay men and lesbians were the result of living in a hostile society where they were relentlessly persecuted. This work too went all but unnoticed for years.

Five years after Hooker's original article, a group of psychoanalysts published a book that tried to provide scientific underpinnings to the psychoanalytic theory of male homosexuality.[17] The authors attempted to apply statistical methods to data collected by distributing questionnaires to psychoanalysts. The analysts had been asked several hundred questions about their patients, including detailed questions about the patient's family, and the authors asked them to draw conclusions about the "closeness" and "emotional warmth" of father-son and mother-son relationships. The authors drew sweeping conclusions about the "causes" of homosexuality from the results, postulating that an emotionally distant father and overinvolved mother had caused these men to become homosexual. The data were drawn from a group of men receiving intensive psychiatric treatment (most hoping to change their sexual orientation from homosexual to heterosexual) and were gathered by asking their therapists to recall what the patients had told them. Despite this biased methodology, the book was warmly received by the psychiatric establishment. Its senior author, Irving Bieber, was accorded immediate recognition as an expert on homosexuality for work that was so methodologically flawed that its results were meaningless. Unfortunately, political and ideological forces rather than science would dictate the "facts" about homosexuality for years to come.

The Impact of the Kinsey and Hooker Studies

Like those of Karl Heinrich Ulrichs a hundred years earlier, the ideas of Alfred Kinsey and Evelyn Hooker about homosexuality were not taken seriously by their contemporaries. For a thousand years, first the church and then the psychiatric establishment had been instructing society on what was moral and normal in sexual matters, and homosexuality was not on either list. A horror of homosexuals was so deeply embedded in theological, legal, and medical theory that questioning the validity of these attitudes was regarded as outrageous and absurd. But like other scientific pioneers, Kinsey and Hooker had blazed a trail that others would follow. Kinsey and Hooker had been behavioral scientists tabulating characteristics of normal individuals, not physicians reporting on disturbed individuals who had come for treatment. Rather than looking for cases of unhappy or disturbed homosexuals among inmates of mental hospitals and prisons, they had applied legitimate scientific methods to the study of sexuality in nonclinical populations. Their methods and the results they had obtained challenged future researchers to find "normal" homosexual individuals for research rather persons in prisons or undergoing treatment for psychiatric problems. As more and more took up this challenge, the study of homosexuality became more unbiased and truly scientific views of homosexuality began to appear, views very different from those presented by Krafft-Ebing and by the Freudians. In the second part of this book we will explore these new views and the work that has produced it.

Sexual Biology

Several years ago, the bright, pretty face of an infant appeared on the cover of one of the major weekly newsmagazines with a headline posing the question "Is This Baby Gay?" Inside was an article titled "Is Homosexuality Born or Bred?"[1] New findings from the field of biology have raised anew an old question about human behavior, this time in relation to sexual orientation. Several of the chapters in the foregoing sections touch on this issue, a tension between two opposing viewpoints, expressed by the juxtaposition of terms like *nature* versus *nurture* and *essentialism* versus *constructionism*.

Thomas Aquinas and other early religious writers declared sodomy a sin anyone might be tempted to commit, not the characteristic of a particular type of person. Karl Heinrich Ulrichs maintained the opposite, writing that men who loved men and women who loved women represented a completely different type of human being, a "third sex" related to, but distinct from, ordinary men and women. Richard Krafft-Ebing lumped "antipathic sexuality" together with a whole variety of aberrations of sexual behavior and thought of it as one possible outcome of worldly stress on a neuropathic disposition. Havelock Ellis, on the other hand, wondered if "sexual inversion" was inborn, the result of a deviation in sexual development which was a permanent attribute of the afflicted. Freud seems to have straddled the fence, even to have taken both positions simultaneously, speaking of "inborn tendencies" and psychosexual development working together to determine "object choice" and sexual orientation. Kinsey conceptualized human sexuality on a continuum and believed that the individual's position along the scale was determined by cultural circumstances, social forces, and even personal choice. Evelyn Hooker considered the "overt homosexual" so obvious a category that she did not even define what she meant by the term in her research papers—to her the idea that certain persons were "homosexual" was self-evident.

Even "before homosexuality" these dichotomies are faintly discernible. For the ancient Greeks, the idea that homosexuality was an individual attribute wasn't at all compelling; they had no word for "homosexuality" or for "a homosexual person." In this ancient culture, many men enjoyed sexual intimacy with other men; the fact that some preferred it much more than others was hardly noticed. Nevertheless, the Greeks invented a story that accounted for essential differences in sexual orientation among individuals: Aristophanes' tale of the "double" creatures—double male, double female, and male-female—which Zeus split "like a hard-boiled egg with a hair" to make new creatures that were either heterosexual or homosexual.

In contrast to the relaxed and accepting attitudes of the ancient Greeks, many later societies discouraged same-sex intimacy, and some severely punished homosexuality. Even in these societies, there seems to have existed some irreducible percentage of persons drawn to same-sex partners for intimacy no matter how awful the penalty.

The idea that there is something essentially different—sexually different—about homosexual individuals recurs again and again throughout history. Philosophers and scientists invented the labels and explanations for the feelings, activities, and relationships that have been presented in the preceding pages: sodomite, Urning, invert, antipathic sexuality, contrary sexual, and finally homosexual—all categories trying to capture the quality and nature of the essence that underlies same-sex intimacy. Individuals such as Karl Ulrichs, John Addington Symonds, and Radclyffe Hall described their inner experience of homosexuality as the process of discovering a force within themselves. Over the next 150 years, thousands more would tell the same story: a gradual unfolding of a sexual life oriented toward persons of their own sex which is compelling and passionate and emotionally fulfilling— and which is no different from that described by persons oriented toward the opposite sex. For most people, this orientation does not change over time but is a personal attribute, an essence arising spontaneously from within them according to the same timetable that governs heterosexual development.

With this idea in mind, we might view the past somewhat differently and not be surprised to find that there have always been homosexual persons—even before the word *homosexuality* existed. Because of complex social factors, these individuals express their sexual orientation differently in each culture. A homosexual person might look different in different cultures. Among the Greeks, the existence of homosexuality has been described as being "submerged within cultural mores."[2] Those for whom same-sex intimacy was consistently and compellingly more satisfying than heterosexual relationships did not stand out from the majority. For most ancient Greeks, perhaps, homosexual intimacy was merely a pleasant sensual diversion from what they experienced as "the real thing": heterosexual intimacy. Among the pre-Columbian native peoples of America, homosexual individuals became berdaches and Amazons—or were killed if the native people happened to be Aztecs. In our time, twenty-five hundred years of cultural shifts have resulted in a world different from those inhabited by the Greeks or the berdache, or for that matter the Urning or the invert. Consequently, we have invented new words and new categories.

The idea of a "sexual essence" challenges those interested in human behavior to describe its nature and discover what biologists call its substrate, the physical substance on which and in which it exists— hormonal systems, chromosomes, the brain. Many researchers are looking for this substrate, persuaded that sexual orientation can be appreciated as a biological as well as a psychological or behavioral phenomenon.

Understanding homosexuality seems necessary for the complete understanding of more basic scientific questions as well. As we will see in this section, geneticists and neuroscientists are studying sexual orientation in order to shed light on a variety of issues in their fields. Scientists have turned to the study of homosexuality as the "exception that proves the rule"—the exception, or variation, that tests a hypothesis about inheritance, about the links between sexuality and brain structure, or about behavioral psychology.

Social forces demand answers to the "nature/nurture" question as well. Religious groups condemn gay men and lesbians for their sinful, immoral "choice" to indulge in same-sex intimacy and fight to keep information about gay people out of schools so as not to "corrupt" children. The National Association for Research and Therapy of Homosexuality purports to "treat" and "cure" homosexuals. American historian John Boswell has stated that "'homosexual/heterosexual' is the . . . foundation of all modern discourse about sexuality—scientific, social, and ethical—and it seems urgent, intuitive and profoundly important to most Americans."[3] A more thorough understanding of what homosexuality is and isn't will inevitably lead to a more rational and humane discourse in our society on the issue. In the next chapters, current research into the biological nature of sexual orientation will be reviewed, work that explores the essence of one of the most basic of human experiences—sexuality.

SEVEN

Sexual Biology I

In the last few years, there has been an explosion of scientific studies on biological factors and sexual orientation. Studies on heredity and brain structure and even studies on seemingly unrelated matters like left-handedness and fingerprint patterns in homosexual men and women have appeared in scientific journals. For many, these studies are the most interesting but also the most difficult to understand sources of new information on homosexuality. There is also information on the biology of sexual orientation which is not so new—studies from the 1970s and even the 1960s which looked at hormones and sexual orientation and discovered some very interesting things.

In this and the next two chapters, we'll delve into all of this—but to be able to understand it all, we'll start with a (short, I promise) biology lesson.

Sexual Development

In the early stages of the development of the human fetus, the two sexes are indistinguishable. In addition, human embryos are quite similar in their very earliest stages of development to the embryos of pigs, chickens, and even fish. It was this observation—that the human fetus doesn't look particularly human at first—which laid to rest the eighteenth-century theory of "preformation," the idea that the organism is fully formed in the egg (ovum) or in the sperm and that development is simply a process of growth (or more precisely, enlargement). With the invention of more and more powerful microscopes, it became apparent to nineteenth-century embryologists that fetal development is a gradual transformation of a single cell, the fertilized egg, into an increasingly complex structure that resembles simple, more primitive organisms at first and only gradually becomes more and more elaborated and complicated and more human. During development, the human embryo passes through stages during which its internal and external anatomy, the structure of its various organs, closely resembles that of more primitive organisms.

The genital area of the human embryo of about six weeks has a series of tubes opening onto the body surface—no external sex organs have yet developed. As in simpler organisms, in both the female and male human embryo the gonads (the organs that will eventually produce sex cells—ova and sperm—the ovaries and testes) are at first located inside the abdominal cavity. A ridge of tissue in the embryo's abdomen will give rise to either ovaries, which will remain inside the abdomen of the female, or testes, which will push out through the abdominal wall during development into a sac that will develop outside the abdominal cavity: the scrotum.

In the human female embryo, the tubes from gonad to body surface (called the Müllerian ducts, after the anatomist who first described them) develop into the organs of the female reproductive system: the fallopian tubes, uterus, and inner portion of the vagina. In the male, these tubes will degenerate. Instead, a different set of tubes grow and become the ducts and organs of the male reproductive system. The details of what tube becomes which duct are not as important as the fact that the precursors of the reproductive organ systems of *both* sexes are present in the embryo of *each*. Early in their development, male embryos have female structures and female embryos have male structures.

The external genitalia of both male and female also develop from a single set of precursor structures present in both sexes. The penis and clitoris both develop from the *genital tubercle*. The same folds of tissue which will form the labia minora in the female will instead elongate and fuse together in the male to form the scrotum.

At the end of the nineteenth century, these details of embryonic development, specifically the fact that human embryos have precursor tissues of the opposite sex's genitalia, were being discovered for the first time. The term *bisexual potential* was being used in the scientific literature and caught the attention of Karl Ulrichs, Havelock Ellis, and, later, Sigmund Freud. Each of these men saw in these discoveries a potential explanation for homosexuality. Ulrichs discussed his belief in a "physical germ" and a "spiritual germ" for sexual functioning in a letter to an uncle in 1862.[1] Later in his pamphlets, he postulated that the Urning had the masculine "male germ" and the female "spiritual germ," the "female spirit in the male body."[2] Havelock Ellis put it this way in *Sexual Inversion*:

> It may be said that at conception the organism is provided with about 50 per cent of male germs and about 50 per cent of female germs, and that as development proceeds either the male or the female germs assume the upper hand, killing out those of the other sex, until in the maturely developed individual only a few aborted germs of the opposite sex are left. In the homosexual person . . . we may imagine that the process has not proceeded normally, on account of some peculiarity in the number or character of either the original male or female germs, or both.[3]

Freud saw fetal bisexuality as evidence of a universal bisexual potential for sexual orientation which early experiences molded into either "normal" or "inverted" sexuality.[4]

Discoveries in the fields of endocrinology and genetics suggested a number of candidates for the various "germs," but in the 1940s, a remarkable discovery about embryonic sexual differentiation was made. Microsurgical techniques had made it possible to remove the developing testes or ovaries from animal embryos without interfering with the rest of their development. It was discovered that removing the embryonic testes from a male embryo caused it to develop female sexual organs—but that removing the ovaries from a female embryo did not interfere with the development of the other female sex organs and genitalia. In other words, some factor produced by the fetal testis is necessary for the development of male organs—if this factor is not present, the organism will develop female organs. Modern embryology has shown that a female principle is dominant in prenatal development; unless something is added, the something being testicular tissue, female anatomy develops.

What does the testis do that makes the embryo develop male organs? Part of what it does, as you might guess, is secrete the male hormone testosterone. (A hormone is a chemical signal released by a gland into the bloodstream to bring about some effect throughout the body.) However, more than testosterone is necessary for male structures to develop. Remember that sexual ducts called the Müllerian ducts develop into the female sex organs in female embryos but wither and regress in males. Testosterone alone is not enough to make this regression happen. Another chemical with the unimaginative but apt title "Müllerian-inhibiting hormone" (MIH) must be present for this regression to occur. Experiments have shown that after a certain point, the development of the Müllerian ducts into female organs cannot be halted by MIH. This illustrates the very important concept of the *critical period* in development: certain developmental processes driven or regulated by hormones (or other factors) must receive their input during a critical period for the regulation or modulation of the process to occur—once the critical period has passed, a kind of "point of no return" is also passed, and the organism is permanently committed along a certain pathway. If a male embryo is castrated *after* the critical period for development of the male sex ducts has passed, an incomplete but distinctively male anatomy results, and the animal will not develop female organs.

By the late 1940s, it had become clear that there is a gene on the "male," or Y, chromosome which is responsible for the development of an embryo into a male. (Remember that there are two human sex chromosomes, the X and Y chromosomes; females have two Xs, males have one X and one Y.) This gene is called the "testis determining factor" (TDF). As it turns out, when this gene switches on early in development, it causes the undifferentiated embryonic gonad to start developing into the testis. When this happens, a whole cascade of events is triggered: the testis starts to secrete MIH and testosterone; these circulating hormones cause one set of the primitive sex ducts to regress and the other to develop into the internal male sex ducts, and the external genital precursors develop into the penis and scrotum. The development of all of the physical aspects of being male is set into motion, including the shape of the pelvis, musculature, and—very important to this discussion—certain aspects of brain development. If the embryo does not have TDF, the gonads develop into ovaries and an alternative cascade of events occurs: the differentiation of female internal and external sex organs, the determination of pelvic shape, and the development of breast tissue and other female characteristics.[5]

If problems in this process of differentiation occur, various medical conditions result from the missteps and defects in the developmental process. It will be useful to review some of these conditions because they provide a great deal of information about the biology of sexuality.

"Androgen insensitivity syndrome" is the result of an inherited defect in the receptor molecule for testosterone. Like other hormones, testosterone in the bloodstream must combine with a receptor on the surface of a cell in order to have its effect. The analogy often used for chemical signals in the body like hormones is that of a key and a keyhole—the key (hormone) must fit into the keyhole (the receptor) in order for the door to open. Individuals with this syndrome have a defective testosterone "keyhole." Therefore, the testosterone produced by their testes has no effect on any of the target tissues. When these individuals are born, they have female genitalia—because the testosterone signal was never received by any of the usual tissues during development. Because the testes normally produce some estrogen as well as testosterone, these individuals develop female breasts and body contours at puberty. Since they have normal female genitalia, they are naturally raised as girls by their parents. Their "true" sex is usually not discovered until they are young adults, when they come for a medical evaluation because of a failure to menstruate or for an infertility evaluation. Studies of the sexual orientation of these women (to all appearances, they *are* women) have found that they are sexually attracted to men. This raises an interesting question: are they "homosexual"? After all, they are genetic males who are attracted to males— once again, the realities of nature confound the categories created by science.

Another sexual "reversal" caused by a genetic defect is congenital adrenal hyperplasia (CAH; also called congenital virilizing adrenal hyperplasia). The adrenal glands, present in both males and females and located above the kidneys, produce a variety of important hormones (cortisol is one) which regulate blood pressure, sugar metabolism, and other important functions. The adrenal glands also produce testosterone—in males *and* females (normally in much smaller amounts than the testes do). CAH occurs when an abnormal enlargement of the adrenal glands or some other genetic defect causes them to secrete an abnormally large amount of testosterone. These high levels of circulating adrenal testosterone during embryonic development cause genetic females with this syndrome to develop masculinized genitalia. (Genetic males are relatively unaffected.) This masculinization ranges from an enlargement of the clitoris to the development of a male-sized penis and fusion of the labia to form a scrotum. A variety of in-between states have been observed as well, which seem to depend on the amount and timing of the excess testosterone. At birth, the external genitalia of genetic females with this syndrome may be ambiguous—it may be genuinely impossible to decide by inspection alone whether the sex organ is a large clitoris or a small penis, whether the child has an incompletely fused scrotum or partially fused labia.

In the 1960s, Dr. John Money of the Johns Hopkins University studied these children in order develop a system for sex assignment for them—which of them would have the best chances of being healthy and happy as boys, which as girls? Previously, they had often been assigned according to a "best guess" based on the masculinity or femininity of their genitalia. Money helped determine that genetic females with this syndrome almost always did better as females—their genetic sex. Adrenogenital children born with a penis-sized clitoris and labia fused into a scrotum now have surgery to feminize their external genitalia, and they are reared as females. Administering steroid medication turns off the abnormal testosterone production in these children and allows their ovaries to function normally. The most interesting finding for the purposes of this discussion is that long-term follow-up studies of girls with CAH found that many of them were "tomboys," high-energy girls with an interest in sports and outdoor activities and fewer daydreams of becoming wives and mothers than their peers. In at least one study, carried into adulthood, a slightly greater than expected number of these girls had become lesbians—sexually attracted to other women as adults. Since these women had been treated for their abnormal hormone levels from infancy, they had normal female levels of estrogen and testosterone throughout their lives. It has been suggested that the higher-than-expected frequency of homosexuality in these women is due to the higher-than-normal levels of testosterone present during their development.[6] These findings point to the possibility that in addition to the developing sex organs, prenatal hormone levels might affect the developing brain as well.

Another group of individuals exposed to abnormal hormone levels during pregnancy were children whose mothers were treated with the synthetic hormone diethylstilbestrol (DES) during pregnancy. During the 1940s and 1950s, DES and other synthetic hormones were administered to women with a history of miscarriage to "shore up" deficiencies of the placental hormones needed to sustain pregnancy until term. (DES turned out to increase the chances of cancer developing in persons whose mothers had been treated with it during their pregnancies, and its use has been abandoned.) The study of these individuals is revealing about the effect of hormones on sexual development because DES is very similar to testosterone but has no significant effect on the development of the sex organs—it affects only the brain. These individuals can be thought of as having had *only their nervous systems* exposed to high testosterone levels during development. In a follow-up study of females who had been exposed to DES during development, a definite increase of homosexual and bisexual fantasy and behavior was noted. Although the numbers of women available for study were small, the percentages are impressive. In one report, 25 percent of the DES-exposed women considered themselves lesbian or bisexual—perhaps ten times the expected rate.[7]

Perhaps the most intriguing of these conditions is a genetically determined hormonal problem called 5-alpha-reductase deficiency syndrome. In this syndrome, genetic males lack an enzyme necessary for normal development of the external genitalia (5-alpha-reductase is the enzyme that converts testosterone to a slightly different form of the hormone necessary for normal development of the penis and scrotum). These genetic males have normal testicular tissue and normal testosterone levels—but at birth they have genitalia that appear to be female. Therefore they are raised by their families as girls. At puberty, however, their testes begin to secrete the usual high levels of testosterone, and these "girls" seem to change into boys. Their voices deepen, their muscles and body fat distribution take on a masculine pattern, and their "clitoris" enlarges into a penis-sized organ.

When a large cluster of persons with this syndrome in the Dominican Republic was studied during the 1970s, it was observed that most of the affected individuals—despite having been raised as girls—adopted a male self-identity at puberty and became erotically oriented toward females. These observations have been interpreted as indicating that male gender identity and heterosexuality are determined prenatally by exposure of the brain to testosterone (remember that these individuals have normal testosterone levels) and that this effect cannot be "overridden" by rearing an individual as a female.[8]

These rare syndromes help us to understand homosexuality because they serve to challenge our usual sexual categories, not only the homosexual/heterosexual dichotomy but the male/female dichotomy as well. Individuals with the androgen insensitivity syndrome are genetic males who look and act like and consider themselves to be females. This syndrome illustrates that individuals' genetic sex can differ from their anatomic sex and from their gender identity (the individual's self-identity as a man or as a woman).

Study of individuals with 5-alpha-reductase deficiency seems to indicate that gender self-identity can differ from *social* gender identity. Being born with feminized genitalia and raised as a girl doesn't prevent a male self-identity and an erotic interest in females from developing in these persons—perhaps because of "masculinization" of the brain.

The "tomboy" behavior and higher-than-expected incidence of homosexuality in females with CAH and females whose mothers were treated with DES during pregnancy have been taken to indicate that high levels of testosterone affect brain development and may cause differences in the pattern of sexual and nonsexual gender role behavior.

It is very important to point out that not all individuals affected by these syndromes show the same pattern of variation in their sexual behavior. Not all CAH females—not even most of them—become lesbians. The same is true for DES-exposed women. Some individuals with 5-alpha-reductase deficiency have been surgically and hormonally treated to prevent pubertal masculinization and prefer to live as females. Studies of individuals with these hormonal abnormalities nevertheless indicate that prenatal hormonal states exert at least some influence on sexual behavior in adulthood.

The study of these rare syndromes, as interesting and useful as it may be, has yielded only incomplete information about the influence of prenatal hormonal events on the brain. Animal studies, however, allow the opportunity to manipulate prenatal hormonal events artificially under controlled conditions. Such studies have complemented and greatly expanded the information gathered from human studies.

The Sexual Brain

In the discussion of the development of the reproductive system earlier in this chapter, the point was made that during embryonic development, simple structures that resemble the organs of simpler types of organisms form the basis for the more complicated structures of the fully developed human anatomy. This principle also governs the development of the most complex and most human of our bodily organs, the brain. The fully developed human brain can also be understood as containing levels of organization in its structure, ranging from simple to astoundingly complex, which parallel and illustrate our evolutionary development. We'll have another short biology lesson here.

At the lowest and simplest level of the human nervous system are the reflexes of the spinal cord which operate simple relay circuits not very different from the primitive nervous system of the earthworm. If you have ever had the experience of accidentally touching a hot stove, you may have noticed that you pull your hand away even before experiencing pain. The sensing of the tissue-damaging heat and the initiation of the muscle jerk that pulls your hand back occur at the level of the spinal cord—no brain input is necessary. The pain signal eventually relayed to higher centers and consciously felt is more of an "FYI" signal that will be registered to help prevent similar experiences in the future.

At the top of the spinal cord, several control centers regulate functions like breathing, blood pressure, and body temperature. These centers also operate without input from higher centers in the brain, which explains why persons who have suffered even catastrophic brain damage still can breathe, sustain a heartbeat, and regulate blood pressure and body temperature.

At a higher level of complexity called the *midbrain* are a series of relay centers that serve to process information received from both "lower" and "higher" centers and refine and elaborate simple reflex motions into complicated, coordinated outputs—posture, complex movements like walking, lifting, reaching, and so forth. Animals that have had higher brain areas surgically removed are still capable of behavior as complex as walking a treadmill—but they are "brain dead" for any more complex behaviors or interactions with their environment.

At the very highest level of organization is the *cerebrum*, which is itself organized into levels of complexity. This astonishingly complex structure coordinates the total input: sight, sound, and touch, memories, experiences, and emotions, initiating complicated behaviors in a way that is still very poorly understood. Whether the behavior is moving a piano, playing a piano, or composing a piano sonata, complex behaviors are possible only with an intact cerebrum. In humans, this level of the brain reaches a size and complexity far beyond that of any other animal. During development the human cerebrum grows to

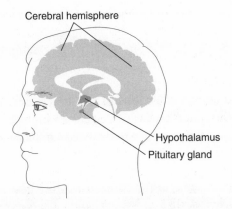

The massive *cerebral hemispheres* envelop "older" areas of the human brain, including the *hypothalamus*, which links the brain to the "master gland," the pituitary.

cover and envelop all the "older" brain areas and even folds in on itself to further enlarge its area and capabilities.

Fairly far down in this hierarchy of control and complexity is a region of the brain called the *hypothalamus*. Literally meaning "beneath the chamber" in Latin, because it forms the lower sides and floor of a liquid-filled brain cavity called the third ventricle, this funnel-shaped structure contains about a teaspoonful of brain tissue. The lower tubelike part of this tiny funnel extends below the surface of the brain and connects with the *pituitary gland*, which sits in an indentation in the floor of the skull whimsically named the *sella turcica* because of its resemblance to a Turkish riding saddle. The hypothalamus occupies a unique position at the interface of the brain and the pituitary gland. The pituitary has been nicknamed the "master gland" because it secretes hormones that regulate many other hormonal systems in the body: the thyroid gland, the adrenal glands, and the gonads: the testes and ovaries.

The structure and function of the hypothalamus are reflected in its key location; like the rest of the brain it has a circuitry of interconnecting neurons that send and receive electrical signals to and from other brain levels—but it also has cells capable of making hormones and releasing them into the bloodstream to send chemical signals to areas of the body with which it has no direct connection. Part brain center and part hormonal regulator, the hypothalamus is thought to translate

one type of information into the other and provide a connection between brain events and hormonal events, the interface where one type
of event interacts with and affects the other. It should come as no
surprise, then, that the hypothalamus, the modulator and translator
between the brain and hormonal systems, contains a number of centers
that are responsible for certain aspects of sexual functioning.

The experiments by which these functions have been demonstrated
have of necessity been performed in laboratory animals, mostly the rat.
In the late 1970s, it was discovered that certain concentrations of brain
cells (such a concentration is called a *nucleus*) in the rat hypothalamus
were involved in sexual behaviors in male and female rats. When a
male rat finds himself in the proximity of a female rat who is in estrus
(the period when the female is fertile and sexually active, sometimes
called being "in heat"), he responds by mounting her back, inserting
his penis, thrusting, and ejaculating his semen. The estrous female,
when stimulated by the male's mounting, crouches, arches her back,
and raises her hindquarters for intercourse, a behavior called *lordosis*.
Mounting and lordosis are very simple, reflexlike behaviors—lordosis
can be triggered in an estrous female simply by touching her hindquarters with a laboratory instrument or technician's finger. Mounting
behavior in the male can also be triggered by a variety of interactions
with other animals, and males will show mounting behavior almost
randomly on occasion, both with nonestrous females and with other
males. Nevertheless, since mounting in males and lordosis in females
occur most often in a sexual situation, and because these mating behaviors are easily observable in the laboratory and easy to quantify (by
simply counting how often the animal exhibits the behavior in question in, say, an hour), they provide good ways to study male and female
sexual behavior in rats.

By surgically destroying various areas of the hypothalamus in rats or
by treating animals with hormones and then observing the effects of
these interventions on the mating reflexes, scientists have discovered
the functions of several areas of the hypothalamus. Surgical destruction of a cluster of cells near the front and center of the hypothalamus
called the *medial preoptic area* (because it is located near the midline of
the hypothalamus and in front of the optic nerves) causes male rats to
lose interest in mating behavior and practically ignore estrous females.
Removing the testes from rats at birth has basically the same effect—
more or less "nonsexual" male rats are produced. When scientists tried

to restore the mating behaviors to the castrated rats by injecting testosterone, something rather odd happened: the male rats showed an increase in *female* mating behavior—lordosis. Further experimentation revealed that for the male rat to be capable of mounting behavior in adulthood, he must have had a certain level of circulating testosterone during a critical period that lasts for about a week after birth. Castrating the rat or administering a drug that interferes with testosterone's effect prevents the development of mounting behavior even if the rat is given "normal" amounts of testosterone by injection later on.[9]

The testosterone is said to have an "organizing effect" on the developing brain, organizing the brain circuits responsible for mounting behavior. After about one week without testosterone, growth and development of the brain has taken another path, and the presence of testosterone after that makes no difference.[10] Anatomic studies of the rat hypothalamus done in the 1970s revealed that one particular nucleus in the preoptic area is larger in male rats than in female. This area has been named the *sexually dimorphic nucleus of the preoptic area* (SDN-POA, or simply SDN) and is believed to be crucial for male mating behavior. It may be that the "mounting circuitry" that testosterone seems to cause is located in the SDN. In male rats castrated at birth, the SDN is the same size as in females.

It would be well to comment here on what these findings in the rat do and do not mean for the study of homosexuality in humans. It has been suggested that these types of experiments provide an "explanation" for human homosexuality. Since a lack of testosterone during a critical period in rat development can cause male rats to exhibit female behaviors, it has been reasoned that a similar lack of testosterone during a critical period of human development causes "a female spirit in a male body," to quote a now familiar early theorist. But it is a speculative leap from female mating behaviors in castrated rats to homosexuality in humans.

It is very important to note that these rat mating behaviors are rather simple reflex behaviors—not unlike the knee-jerk reflex in humans. Animals have a variety of mating, feeding, and offspring-rearing behaviors that are stereotyped and automatic in the extreme; they are usually called "instincts" to distinguish them from similar human behaviors. Although we humans recognize powerful motivations that arise within ourselves which are related to these instincts, our infinitely more complex intellectual and social capabilities usually dominate them. Our immense capacity for behavioral modulations based on language and social development allows us to override many of the instincts still "wired" in some residual way in our brains.

Observations of certain behaviors in a certain species of animal apply only to that animal. Similarities of behavior between different species do not necessarily prove that the underlying phenomena are the same. Several species of birds fly south for the winter, and so do some humans—but the underlying motivations and the hormonal and neurological basis for these behaviors are obviously quite different! Even in the rat, further research has shown that the hormonal influence story is more complicated than it first appeared—it turns out that estrogen levels are important as well for development of mating behaviors. In addition, there may be a "defeminization" process in the rat brain which occurs independently of the testosterone "masculinizing" process.

As with our discussion of the development of the reproductive organs, the details of exactly which hormone does what are not as important as the principle these experiments illustrate: in the rat, sex hormones have effects on the developing nervous system and exert this effect during critical periods. Once the critical period is over, irreversible developmental effects have occurred which may affect later sexual behavior. To discover whether a similar process occurs in the developing human brain, we must first answer a more basic question: Are there differences in the hypothalamic structure between human male and female brains? The answer is yes.

In the late 1980s, the same researchers who had done much of the experimental work with the rat hypothalamus announced that they had discovered several hypothalamic nuclei in the human brain which are also sexually dimorphic—of a different size in men and in women. They had located a group of four previously undescribed neuronal collections in the forward (anterior) section of the human hypothalamus and named them *interstitial nuclei of the anterior hypothalamus* (INAH). Each nucleus is further designated by number: INAH 1, INAH 2, INAH 3, and INAH 4. INAH 2 and INAH 3 were described as being dimorphic, different between the sexes. The size differences in INAH 2 seemed related to age more than to sex, but the INAH 3 was unequivocally larger in men than in women.[11]

I won't keep those readers in suspense who already know where this discussion is leading—to Simon LeVay's 1991 study comparing the size of hypothalamic nuclei in gay men and in nongay men. Yes, it was the INAH 3, the sexually dimorphic nucleus, which Dr. LeVay discovered to be smaller in gay men than in nongay men. This was the first structural brain difference between homosexual and heterosexual men ever described. But before examining that study and discussing its implications, other aspects of the sexual development of the brain need to be touched upon.

Beyond the Hypothalamus

Women and men differ in many ways above and beyond their anatomy and reproductive physiology. Socialization and cultural determinants are responsible for many, perhaps most, of these differences, but certain differences in temperament, social patterns, and even intellectual skills appear to be innate. Some of these differences between males and females even seem to extend across species. One of these is in an area of childhood behavior called "rough and tumble play."

Little boys are more active as a rule than little girls. Scientists have noticed this pattern in other animals as well, including rats and hamsters, monkeys and apes, and even in sheep. In humans, the pattern has been called an "energy expenditure" difference, with a typical expression being outdoor games and sports. In animals, the comparable type of behavior has been called "play-fighting" because the animals wrestle and snarl and nip each other. Although this is the sort of playing commonly observed in puppies and kittens, these household animals show no sexual dimorphism—males and females show the behavior in equal amounts. In the rats and monkeys, however (and humans, too, for that matter), males and females both show play-fighting, but the males engage in it much more often than the females.

In rats, it has been shown that this behavioral pattern is under the control of testosterone and appears to depend on a certain level of testosterone being present during the same critical period during which mounting behavior "circuitry" is being organized: the first week or so after birth. If male rats are castrated at birth, they show no more play-fighting than females. If females are exposed to testosterone, their play is as rough and tumble as males. The same phenomenon has been demonstrated in rhesus monkeys, except that the critical period in this species occurs before birth. In addition, although female mon-

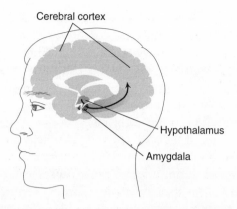

Cerebral cortex

Hypothalamus

Amygdala

The almond-shaped *amygdala* shares connections with the *hypothalamus* and radiates connecting fibers through the limbic system (*arrow*) into the *cerebral cortex*.

keys exposed to testosterone before birth play-fight more than other females, they do not fight as much as males.

In both the rat and the monkey, the brain structure believed likely to play a key role in play-fighting is the *amygdala*—a small collection of cells that share connections with the hypothalamus. (The amygdala is shaped like an almond in humans; its name comes from the Greek word for almond.) Several collections of cells in the amygdala have been shown to be of different sizes in male and female animals of several species. The amygdala forms part of a complex set of connections between the hypothalamus and the cerebral cortex called the *limbic system.* Just as the hypothalamus is the interface of the brain and the master gland, the limbic system, a series of structures and connections that rim the inner edges of the cerebral cortex, is the interface of the hypothalamus and the cerebral cortex. The word *limbus* means "margin" or "border" and is descriptive of the limbic system's location.

Remember that the cerebral cortex is the massively complex structure responsible for the "highest," most complicated functions of the nervous system, where consciousness resides. It is thought that the limbic system is where emotion resides, anger, joy, fear—and perhaps love. It is one of the most poorly understood areas of the entire nervous system. In humans, destruction of important areas of the limbic system by a tumor or stroke results in various clinical syndromes often characterized by a loss of emotional responsiveness, leaving victims listless, apathetic—and usually totally uninterested in sex. In monkeys, surgical destruction of the amygdala area of the limbic system does not make them lose interest in sex but instead causes a syndrome that includes, among other symptoms, a total absence of sexual "directiveness" such that they sexually approach other animals of either sex and even try to mate with inanimate objects.

Again, the details of the anatomy and physiology are not as important as the observation that experiments with animals have determined that *hormonal events* during a *critical period* cause changes in a behavior that differs between male and female individuals (rough and tumble play). This is probably because these events have an *organizing effect* on brain structures known to be involved with sexual behavior and aggression in animals—and probably in humans as well.

Earlier in this chapter the clinical syndrome "congenital adrenal hyperplasia" was described: a genetic defect that causes higher-than-normal levels of testosterone to circulate in the developing fetus. Remember that studies of females with this syndrome showed that they were more likely to report "tomboy" behavior; this, of course, is "rough and tumble play" and suggests that this behavior may have determining factors similar to those that have been demonstrated in the rat—prenatal hormonal events.

If certain hormonal events have been shown to increase "rough and tumble play" in human females, what about boys who show less-than-expected "rough and tumble play" during their childhood? Focused studies of "rough and tumble play" in boys do indeed turn out to be revealing about sexual behavior in adulthood.

An interesting and complicated side issue springs from the fact that while "tomboy" behavior in girls is not particularly singled out for concern, "sissy" behavior among boys is. A moment's reflection on the connotations of the words *tomboy* and *sissy* makes plain the tremendously different values placed on cross-gender behavior in males versus in females—a reflection of the relative value placed on masculine versus feminine behavior by our society. "Tomboy" behavior in girls is frequently dismissed as "a phase," but in boys, a preference for quiet pastimes, nonaggressive social play, or feminine behaviors provokes alarm in parents and contempt among peers—undoubtedly because of the popular stereotype of the "sissy" boy who becomes homosexual in erotic orientation as he gets older. As with many stereotypes, this one is not entirely accurate, but it has some basis in fact nonetheless. The validity of this idea—that decreased "rough and tumble play" during childhood predicts homosexuality in adulthood—has been examined in two ways, through retrospective study and prospective study.

Retrospective study of the issue involves asking adults about childhood experiences. In studies in which homosexual men have been asked about their childhood experiences, the results clearly support the idea that *gender-discordant behavior* in childhood (behavior more like that expected of the opposite sex than one's own) has some predictive value for adult sexual behavior. A large study of the sexual development of men and women conducted during the 1970s revealed that almost half of the men who identified themselves as homosexual recalled less interest in sports and outdoor activities and more interest in quiet, solitary activities such as reading, music, or art.[12]

Retrospective studies are subject to many confounding factors, most notably the fallibility of human memory. A more subtle but very powerful source of error is the tendency of people to remember things in a way that helps them make sense of their lives. Remembrances of events are colored by emotional meaning, sometimes distorted by the desire for their story to be consistent, logical, and reasonable—in some cases, perhaps, by the desire to fulfill the expectations of the interviewer. Another problem with any study of group attributes and behaviors is the possibility that the group studied is not really representative of the group one wishes to study. Sometimes the way one recruits individuals for a study overloads the study group with a particular subtype of individuals, a phenomenon called "ascertainment bias." Are gay men who are willing to participate in a study truly representative of homosexual males?

Prospective studies avoid some of these pitfalls. A prospective study involves studying subjects over time to see if the predictions the model makes turn out to be accurate. This type of study is fiendishly difficult to do because it involves such a huge time commitment—keeping track of individuals for years, sometimes for decades. Nevertheless, several researchers have followed boys identified during childhood as having play patterns different from those of their peers as they matured into adulthood. These studies followed boys who strongly avoided sports and rough and tumble play and preferred to play with dolls. Not only was their social play primarily with girls, but they engaged in cross-dressing play and in role-play as girls. These boys represented the extreme as far as cross-gender behavior—the studies were carried out at mental health facilities on boys so gender-discordant that their parents had sought psychological evaluation for them. This is certainly a serious ascertainment bias if one wants to extrapolate the results to all males. Nevertheless, the results are so striking and unequivocal that they bear examination.

In the most carefully done of these studies,[13] two groups of boys were studied for up to fifteen years from an average age of 7½ years to between the ages of 13 and 23. The study group (forty-four boys) had been brought by their parents for evaluation of cross-gender behavior, and the control group (fifty-six boys) was a recruited sample of paid volunteers. The subjects were interviewed regularly over the years of the study, and at the conclusion, the mental health professionals interviewing the subjects as older adolescents and young adults asked them questions about sexual behavior, erotic dreams, and masturbation fantasies in order to rate each on the 0 to 6 Kinsey scale. Almost half of the "sissy" boys received a Kinsey score of 5 or 6 (predominantly or exclusively homosexual) as young adults. All of the control group scored 0 or 1 (predominantly or exclusively heterosexual). Just as interesting as the striking increase in homosexual orientation in the gender-discordant boys is the fact that *not all* of them had high Kinsey scores. Even though the study group represented the extreme as far as decreased rough and tumble play, many of these boys scored 0 or 1 on the Kinsey scale as young adults. This study provides a strong indication that there is a link between childhood play behavior and adult sexual orientation, but as with other studies in humans looking at the link between homosexuality and practically anything, nothing is 100 percent, and substantial numbers of subjects do not show the expected pattern—in this study, twelve of the young men who had shown extreme cross-gender behavior as children reported exclusively heterosexual orientation in fantasy and behavior.

Is there any evidence that rough and tumble play in humans is influenced by hormone levels during development as it is in other animals? Animal studies would predict that testosterone levels in the body during a critical period before birth bring about rough and tumble play through a masculinizing effect on the brain. Is there an "experiment of nature," a clinical syndrome in humans, in which males have lower-than-usual levels of testosterone during development?

There is one that may be close, called XXY syndrome (also known as

Kleinfelter's syndrome). As the name of the syndrome indicates, persons with this syndrome have an extra copy of the X chromosome, the "female" chromosome. The effect of the extra X during early life appears to be minimal: these individuals have normal male sexual organs and normal testosterone levels during childhood, although for reasons that are unclear, they tend to be taller than average and have lower-than-average IQ scores. At puberty, their testes start to degenerate and testosterone levels drop. They frequently have breast enlargement, they have smaller-than-average genitalia, and their body shape is described as "eunuchoid"—having a femalelike fat distribution. Early studies seemed to indicate that a variety of serious psychological problems invariably accompanied this chromosomal abnormality. However, the subjects of these studies came from clinic samples and institutions, another example of ascertainment bias. In the late 1980s, an ambitious team of American and Danish researchers set out to overcome this ascertainment bias problem by looking for XXY men in the *general* population to interview. With remarkable thoroughness and sheer persistence, they were able to do chromosomal analyses on an astonishing 90 percent of the men born in Copenhagen between 1944 and 1947 who were over six feet tall (remember that XXY men are taller than average). They tested 4,139 men altogether and found 16 with the extra X chromosome, of whom 14 agreed to participate in the study, undergoing interviews, psychological testing, and blood tests for hormone levels.

Several interesting discoveries were made. First, only two men had lower-than-normal testosterone levels, and the average level of all the men was in the normal range. Two reported having fathered children. No particular pattern of psychological problems was found. As far as sexual behavior, these men had a decreased interest in sex compared with a control group. They were older when they had their first sexual intercourse, had intercourse less often, and reported fewer partners— two were still virgins. They also reported significantly less interest in boys' games as children and significantly more homosexual contacts than the control group.[14]

These results seem to indicate that the extra X chromosome decreased childhood masculine behavior (rough and tumble play) and also led to a decreased amount of sexual behavior in adulthood. The mechanism of this effect does not seem to involve testosterone: these XXY men had fairly normal testosterone levels. Although there were increased homosexual contacts, the subjects' generally low interest in sex makes the significance of this unclear (the authors did not give Kinsey ratings on the subjects). Does a decreased testosterone effect on the brain during a critical period during development explain the findings? One might speculate that the extra X chromosome somehow interferes with the effect of testosterone. Do these results show a link between decreased rough and tumble play during childhood and lower-than-average testosterone levels? Perhaps; but the link is speculative at best. The link to adult homosexuality is even more flimsy.

A much stronger link between prenatal hormones and rough and tumble play in males is found in boys whose mothers were exposed to masculinizing hormones during pregnancy. Like DES, 19-nor-17-alpha-ethynyl-testosterone (mercifully abbreviated 19-NET) is similar to progesterone, the hormone secreted by the placenta to sustain pregnancy. But, as the last four syllables of its full name indicate, 19-NET is related to testosterone. Female 19-NET children sometimes had masculinized genitals at birth, but it is the psychological and behavioral profiles of the boys exposed to 19-NET before birth which are the most interesting findings.

One laboratory studied several 19-NET boys with brothers who had *not* been exposed to the hormone[15]—an almost perfect control subject for the boy being studied, since brothers are genetically similar and have similar home environments. The researchers found "consistent and robust differences in physical aggression scores" between 19-NET boys and their brothers. Boys of various ages from young children to college students were studied. The 19-NET boys were more assertive and competitive than their brothers. The 19-NET females showed more physical aggressiveness than their unexposed sisters. These data support the view that rough and tumble play in humans is strongly determined by prenatal testosterone levels.

It is not difficult to get lost in all this data about hormones and brain nuclei. But for all this complexity, these studies illustrate a few points that are not difficult to grasp: Male and female sex organs develop from the same embryonic tissues. Exposure to hormones during development determines whether male or female organs develop. In animals, laboratory experiments indicate that the *brain* is affected by hormonal levels as well and that sexual behavior during adulthood depends to some extent on hormonal events during development.

Humans who were exposed to abnormal hormone levels during their development because of rare medical conditions show differences in how "rough and tumble" they are as children, a behavior that has been linked to sexual orientation in adulthood. Some studies suggest that the abnormal hormone levels to which these individuals are exposed during development make them more likely to be homosexual or bisexual as adults.

The brain centers that are affected by hormonal levels in rats are found in humans as well and are different sizes in men than they are in women. At least one study found that one of these centers was different in a group of gay men compared with a group of heterosexual men.

Taken together, all this work indicates that hormonal levels during development may have an effect on sexual orientation in adulthood. In the next chapter, we'll discuss even more evidence that this is so.

Sexual Biology II

Right Brain—Left Brain

In 1985, a comprehensive three-part article appeared in the medical journal *Archives of Neurology* discussing in detail the phenomenon of "cerebral lateralization"—the organization of different functions of the brain on the two different sides of the cerebrum. The most obvious example of cerebral lateralization in humans is, of course, handedness: the preference of right-hand versus left-hand use. One hand is preferred over the other because one side of the brain is more highly developed for this use than the other. In the article, almost buried among complex and clinical topics like the genetics of handedness and the association between handedness and various learning disabilities, is a short section with the heading "Homosexuality" which begins with the sentence: "Several homosexuals have written to us suggesting that there is a high rate of left-handedness in this population but no study of this has yet been reported."[1]

On the face of it, it would seem that looking for any kind of link between handedness and sexual orientation would be a ludicrous endeavor, reminiscent of the very seriously held theory, referred to by Havelock Ellis in *Sexual Inversion*, that whether or not a man could whistle was highly predictive of whether or not he was homosexual. Which hand a person writes with would seem to have absolutely nothing to do with his or her choice of sexual partners. Nevertheless, several studies indicate that more gay men and lesbians are left-handed than would be expected from the proportion of left-handed persons found in the general population. Psychological research has shown that handedness, as well as other functions of the cerebral hemispheres, differs between men and women (and between male and female members of other species also). These differences might to some extent be determined by, as you might have guessed by now, the level of certain hormones reaching the fetus during embryonic development.

In the previous chapter, we noted that the cerebrum is responsible for the highest levels of functioning of the nervous system. Whereas the more primitive areas of the brain such as the hypothalamus are primarily responsible for managing various inner workings of the body, the cerebrum manages interactions between the individual and his or her environment. Input from the visual, auditory, and other senses is processed, and output such as coordinated movements and speech is organized and initiated. The cerebrum is divided down the middle, front to back, so that it actually consists of two halves that are joined together by a massive collection of connecting fibers, the *corpus callosum* (literally "calloused body" or "hard body," referring to the solid texture the fibers give to this area compared with the soft, almost gelatinlike texture of the outer parts of the cerebrum; see figure on the next page). Brain scientists often speak of "the cerebral hemispheres" rather than of "the cerebrum" to emphasize the fact that this area of the brain, though massively connected, is separated into two matching halves.

Each of the two cerebral hemispheres controls muscle movements on the *opposite* side of the body. Because of the way the visual system works, this "contralateral" organization, though it appears convoluted, turns out to be a most efficient arrangement for organizing movements of the body in response to visual input from the eyes. The left hemisphere controls the right side of the body. Persons who are right-handed are said to be "left-hemisphere dominant" because their left hemisphere is superior to the right in organizing and executing fine motor movements. In 1861, the great pathologist Paul Broca determined that the center for the initiation of speech and language is also located in a specific area (now called "Broca's area" after him) on the left hemisphere.[2] Since Broca's time, more and more information has been gathered about the functions of the cerebral hemispheres, and it has been determined that many functions are lateralized, that is, they

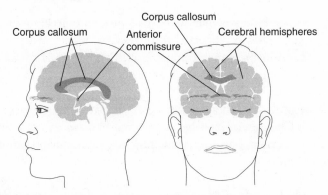

The *corpus callosum* and the *anterior commissure* provide the connecting fibers between each of the two *cerebral hemispheres*.

are predominantly controlled by areas in only one cerebral hemisphere. One of these is visuo-spatial ability—the ability to visualize and analyze three-dimensional space and to control the position and orientation of the body and the limbs in space.

Studies have shown that men and women differ in various psychological abilities.[3] This difference is especially true of abilities that are highly lateralized—abilities that tend to reside more on one side of the brain than on the other. For example, on average, men perform better on tasks of visuo-spatial ability than women. Gender-based differences exist even in lower animals—in the laboratory rat, for example. Male rats learn to run a maze more quickly than female rats and make fewer errors when repeating the run, indicating superior visuo-spatial ability. Removing the gonads of adult rats does not have any effect on performance of either the males or the females, but hormonal treatments shortly after birth do. (Remember that the critical period for many hormonal *organizing* effects on the rat brain is during the neonatal period, shortly *after* birth.) Treatment of neonatal female rats with testosterone improved their learning times; neonatal castration increased the learning time for male rats.[4]

While it might be tempting and certainly interesting to build human-sized mazes and set men and women racing through them, visuo-spatial ability can be measured in humans quite accurately and much more easily with pencil-and-paper tests. The Mental Rotations Test is about the best one available to demonstrate gender differences in visuo-spatial ability. In this test, the subject is shown pictures of complicated three-dimensional objects viewed from different angles and is asked to pick out two views of the same object. This test thus requires the subject to visualize each two-dimensional picture as a three-dimensional object that must then be mentally rotated and compared with other objects.

On average, men perform better than women do on this test. They also do better on tests of target-directed gross motor skills such as guiding or intercepting projectiles—a neuropsychological way of describing most sports. These seem to be right-hemisphere functions. Women test better on a number of language skills, for example, a skill called "ideational fluidity"—the ability to organize ideas and language efficiently. This skill can be measured by asking subjects to list as many words as they can which begin with, say, the letter B, or to list as many objects that are colored red as they can think of in a certain time period. Women are also better at fine complex motor movements requiring precision and pinpoint accuracy, as well as at certain types of visual memory, such as recalling landmarks or objects along a travel route. (Female rats do better in mazes if markers are put in the maze to serve as navigational aids, whereas the addition or removal of navigational markers does not affect the performance of male rats.) Men tend to be better at mathematical reasoning and problem solving, but women excel at fast and accurate computations.

It might be argued that our culture has defined different roles and tasks for men and for women and that these tests are measuring the effects of practice and skill development in socially conditioned categories rather than innate differences in brain function. By testing young children and by asking adults to perform novel, unpracticed behaviors, these effects can be minimized. Most experts agree that differentials in certain skills are indeed a function of brain differences and not merely a reflection of skills learned or acquired along sex-role lines.

Do these differences explain why more women than men do embroidery in their free time and more men than women play golf? Do they explain why some men can't get dressed in the morning without asking their wives for help finding things, or some men's obstinate refusal to stop and ask for directions during a drive? In the last decade or so, women have made better inroads increasing their percentages in the fields of medicine and law than in engineering. Publishers know for a fact that women make up a larger percentage of the book-buying market than men. It's difficult to rule out at least some effect of innate brain differences on behaviors and activities that play on one set of skills or another.

What is the evidence that prenatal hormonal levels cause these differences between the sexes in humans? The rare medical conditions we reviewed in the last chapter seem to verify that hormones have a powerful effect on the development of these sets of skills. Remember that females born with congenital adrenal hyperplasia (CAH) are exposed to higher levels of testosterone prenatally than is normal. Several studies of CAH women reveal that they indeed perform better on average than unaffected women on tests of visuo-spatial ability, tests that seem to measure "masculine" brain functions. Persons with androgen insensitivity syndrome have a defective receptor for testosterone and therefore are exposed to absolutely no testosterone in utero, not even to the testosterone put out by the maternal adrenal glands. Thus they are exposed to even less testosterone during development than normal women. Not only do these individuals perform more poorly on tests of visuo-spatial skills than their male relatives, but they perform more poorly than their female relatives, too.[5]

As a group, men seem to have more lateralization of their brains than women do. Measurements of the thickness of the cerebral cortex on the right versus the left reveal that in male rats the right side (the location of visuo-spatial control) is thicker than on the left. In humans a similar difference has been found in fetal male brains but not in adult men. The fact that women seem less affected than men by strokes affecting the speech center on their speech-dominant hemisphere has been interpreted as indicating that women have more "bilateral" (both-sided) representation of speech. It has been suggested that the higher levels of testosterone present in the male fetus are responsible for the observed greater lateralization in male brains.

It is thought that in males, the same high levels of testosterone which masculinize the external genitalia, the hypothalamus, and other body structures cause an earlier maturing of the right hemisphere. This is thought to solidify in some way the circuitry responsible for visuo-spatial functioning and other "masculine" talents. This would seem to explain the more solid visuo-spatial skills in men and men's greater separation of functions among the two hemispheres—the greater lateralization or functional asymmetry of the male brain. It is also thought to explain the fact that more men than women are left-handed. This theory would predict that lesbians would tend to be left-handed—if their sexual orientation is to some extent steered by higher-than-usual levels of testosterone. This proves to be the case. In one study, 69 percent of the lesbians studied showed left-handedness for writing and other activities, such as brushing their teeth and threading a needle, as compared with 35 percent of the general female population.[6] CAH women are also more likely to be left-handed. Another study showed that gay men are more likely to be left-handed than men are generally,[7] the opposite of what one might predict from a strictly hormonal theory of homosexuality—but other researchers have not reproduced these findings.[8]

What happens during development to cause left-handedness? It is thought that in some individuals the testosterone effect is somehow "dampened" and the two halves of the cerebrum are so similar that handedness and language functions get randomly assigned to either the right or the left side. In some individuals these functions are shared between the two cerebral hemispheres, and "mixed" dominance results. In mixed dominance, both hemispheres participate more or less equally in functions. As it turns out, left-handed persons frequently show mixed dominance. Some left-handers use their left hand to write with a pen but their right hand to write with chalk on a blackboard. The German painter Menzel wrote with his left hand but painted with his right. I myself write left-handed but hold a golf club and baseball bat as right-handers do.

Several studies have demonstrated differences between homosexual and nonhomosexual individuals in brain functions known to be lateralized. Gay men performed less well than nongay men in a study that used the Mental Rotations Test to measure visuo-spatial ability, a result that is in the "expected" direction. However, lesbians perform about the same on these tests as nonlesbian women do, an unexpected finding.[9] In a study that measured the accuracy with which individuals of both sexes and differing sexual orientations could strike a target with a projectile, nongay men did better than gay men, and lesbians performed better than nonlesbian women even when their sports history was factored out.[10] Greater verbal ability in gay men compared with nongay men has been reported, another expected result. But other studies have not found such a difference. In a study of homosexual and nonhomosexual men and women which investigated cerebral lateralization with a sophisticated technique that measures language processing in each cerebral hemisphere (called "linguistic dichotic listening"), functional differences were found in both the gay men and the lesbians compared with the nonhomosexual men and women.[11]

Several studies have claimed to have found anatomic correlates of increased functional symmetry in the brains of gay men—a *structural* difference in brain anatomy of gay men which would indicate more evenly divided brain functions between the two cerebral hemispheres. As noted above, the great majority of fibers connecting the two hemispheres are in the corpus callosum. But there is another bundle of fibers toward the front of the brain called the *anterior commissure* (Latin word for "connection"; see figure, p. 124). This structure is larger in women than in men, possibly because the greater bilateral (two-sided) organization of the female brain requires more interconnecting fibers. If gay men are more "mixed" in their cerebral organization, they would also need more connecting fibers. In 1992, it was reported from autopsy studies that the anterior commissure was larger in the brains of gay men than in nongay men.[12] What is even more striking is that when corrections were made for the fact the overall brain size is greater in men than in women, the average size of the anterior commissure of the gay men was almost exactly the same size as in women. More recently, a study was published in which the size of the corpus callosum, the main connector between the cerebral hemispheres, was measured in live volunteers by MRI scan. It was reported that one section of the corpus callosum was 13 percent larger in a group of gay men than it was in a group of heterosexual men.[13]

In summary, lateralized brain functions such as handedness and visuo-spatial ability which are affected by prenatal hormones have been demonstrated to differ between groups of homosexual men and women and groups of heterosexual men and women. Even more compelling is the finding that the expected brain structures, the cerebral "connectors," the corpus callosum and the anterior commissure, are also found to be different in male homosexuals—larger, as would be predicted.

Gunter Dörner and the "Stress Theory"

Let us pause here for a cautionary tale about the science of sexual orientation, one illustrating the dangers of oversimplification of theory and of jumping too quickly to unwarranted conclusions.

At least one scientist has taken all of the data about prenatal testosterone levels and offered a comprehensive biological theory of male and female homosexuality. Gunter Dörner, a German endocrinologist, has been doing research on hormone levels in animals and humans and using the findings to support a hormonal theory of homosexuality for more than twenty-five years. In a pair of papers published in the late 1960s in the British *Journal of Endocrinology*, he laid the groundwork by duplicating and confirming the experiments with rats which showed that adult mating reflexes are organized by testosterone during a critical period shortly after birth. Dörner's papers, while not presenting any really new information, nevertheless stand out from others on the subject because of their titles: "Induction and Prevention of Male Homosexuality by Androgen" and "Hormonal Induction and Prevention of Female Homosexuality."[14] It is rather a surprise to read the papers and discover that the "homosexuality" Dörner was inducing and preventing was the lordosis reflex in male rats, a phenomenon that he did not hesitate to offer as an animal model of homosexuality in humans. It is one of a number of assumptions that have made Dörner's work controversial and often criticized.

At a conference in Boston in 1993 in which eminent scientists from across the United States gathered to discuss the biological aspects of sexual orientation, Dr. Roger Gorsky, the neuroscientist who just might know more about the rat hypothalamus than anyone else on the planet, discussed these assumptions. He showed a short film of male rats running around a small cage, sniffing each other, twitching their whiskers, and occasionally arching their back. "I invite you to decide what, if anything, *this* has to do with sexual orientation in humans," he said to the scientists gathered in the room. His message was clear: human sexuality is so infinitely more complex than mating reflexes in rats that any comparison of possible underlying physiology can assume only the most general connections between the two phenomena.

Dörner's assumption that the artificial production of the lordosis reflex in male rats is equivalent to human male homosexuality is a tenuous and unvalidated presumption, to say the least. Nevertheless, convinced of the basic validity of the rat model, Dörner started looking for some indication of "feminization" of the hypothalamus in gay men. By 1976, he believed he had found it.

Remember that the hypothalamus is the interface between the brain and the pituitary gland, where the nervous system and the hormonal systems of the body meet and interact. One of the important activities that take place at this interface is the regulation of the menstrual cycle. In women of childbearing age, when an ovum begins to develop in the ovary every month, ovarian tissue begins to secrete estrogen into the bloodstream. This rising estrogen level is monitored by the hypothalamus. When a certain threshold is reached, the hypothalamus signals the pituitary gland to release a pulse of luteinizing hormone (LH). This surge of LH triggers ovulation, the release of the ovum from the ovary. This phenomenon is called a "positive feedback" effect: rising levels of estrogen cause a rise in LH levels. The effect can be artificially produced in human females by giving them an injection of estrogen. The proper dose can "fool" the hypothalamus and cause an LH surge from the pituitary which can be measured. The pituitary of the human male also secretes LH—but for a different purpose. In the male, LH stimulates the production of testosterone by the testes, which in turn stimulates sperm production, among other things. There is also a feedback effect in males between the hypothalamus, the pituitary, and the testes which involves LH, but there is no "pulse" of LH as is seen in females.

In the mid-1970s, Dörner claimed to have demonstrated that an LH surge could be triggered by an injection of estrogen in homosexual males but not in heterosexual males. He concluded that gay men had a "feminized" brain, presumably resulting from abnormally low levels of testosterone during a critical period of fetal brain development.

In later papers he went on to claim that lower-than-normal testosterone levels in the developing fetus could be caused by maternal stress during pregnancy. This idea was derived from experiments that showed that subjecting pregnant female rats to stress, such as by confining them in a plastic tube under bright lights for prolonged periods of time, will lower testosterone levels in male fetuses. The male offspring of the stressed females will show the adult behavioral changes typical of male rats with "feminized" brains: increased lordosis.

Dörner then set about trying to demonstrate a link between human male homosexuality and prenatal maternal stress. In the early 1980s, two papers appeared which purported to do this. In the first, it was claimed that there was a greater-than-expected incidence of homosexuality among men whose mothers were born in Germany during the Second World War, inarguably a time of stress.[15] In the second, mothers of homosexual sons and of nonhomosexual sons were interviewed and asked to recall periods of stress.[16] In this study, mothers of gay sons recalled stressful periods more frequently than mothers of nongay sons.

Almost immediately a storm of protest arose over the scientific validity of Dörner's work—as well as questions regarding his motives for pursuing this line of research. In an editorial that appeared in the scientific journal *Archives of Sexual Behavior*, officers of the German Society for Sexual Research denounced Dörner as trying to "eradicate homosexuality by means of radical endocrine intervention during fetal development."[17] To some extent Dörner brought these charges on himself, referring to higher or lower levels of prenatal testosterone as a "teratogen," a word used to refer to agents that cause birth defects. Dörner denied the society's charge that he was searching for a method of "endocrinological euthanasia" for homosexuals and characterized the editorial as "filled with lies, imputations, defamations and slanders." He admitted, however, that the impetus for his research was "the prevention of hormone . . . disturbances of the brain . . . associated with permanent somatic, mental, and/or psychic disabilities."[18]

Although this theory of male homosexuality appears simple and clear, there are many problems with Dörner's studies. Perhaps the most serious is the inability of other researchers to reproduce the "intermediate" LH surge in gay men in several repeat studies. In addition, animal scientists have pointed out that several species of primates (monkeys and apes) have an LH regulation system in the male which is different from that found in rats, the animal model used for much of Dörner's work. Another study that tested the theory looked at male-to-female transsexuals. The subjects were tested before and after the surgical removal of their testes (part of the sex-change operation). These persons had the "male" LH response to estrogen injection before their testes were removed and the "female" response after.[19] This was interpreted as indicating that whatever variation in LH response is observed in men is related to some factor secreted by the testes—that it has nothing to do with the hypothalamus. Further, female CAH patients who have been exposed to high enough levels of masculinizing hormones to "masculinize" their nervous systems do not have any reproductive abnormalities, whereas Dörner's hormonal theory would predict that they would not ovulate normally.

The "war population" studies are subject to criticism because they attempted to measure rates of homosexuality in men of different age groups and drew their data from public health statistics on men with venereal diseases. The greater incidence of homosexuality Dörner found may only reflect the rates of sexually transmitted disease in homosexual versus nonhomosexual men—or perhaps differences in where homosexual versus nonhomosexual men go to be treated for venereal diseases—rather than the rate of homosexuality in the male population as a whole.

As for the study asking mothers of gay sons to recall stressful events during pregnancy, a more recent study asked mothers who had a gay son and a nongay son to recall stressful events during each pregnancy. Thus each reporter/mother served as her own "control"—the same subject reported on two different pregnancies. These women did not report any excess of stressful events while pregnant with their gay son compared with the pregnancy with their nongay son.

In summary, Gunter Dörner's "stress theory" of homosexuality hasn't held up very well; it is highly questionable that the "LH surge" has any relevance to sexual orientation in humans. There would appear to be a more insidious problem here, as well—Dörner's assumptions about human homosexuality. Dörner's writings indicate that he considered homosexuality a "psychic disability." He even stated that "it might become possible in the future . . . to prevent the development of homosexuality,"[20] a suggestion all the more chilling coming from a German scientist only fifty years after the "scientists" of the Third Reich attempted genetic and prenatal manipulations to rid the "master race" of various "impurities." The lesson here is that too many prior assumptions make for bad science. Good research tries, to quote Kinsey again, "to discover what the facts of the universe are . . . whether they are in conformance with anyone's preconception or no."

Prenatal Hormones and Sexual Orientation

There is so much evidence linking the effects of prenatal hormone levels to adult sexual orientation that one cannot help but be curious as to the nature of the links. Measures of handedness, psychological profile studies, and several anatomic studies of gay men and lesbians reveal a number of brain differences between them and their nongay counterparts. Although understanding these differences to mean that lesbians have a "masculinized" brain and gay men a "feminized" brain is a naive oversimplification, it seems clear that development patterns of brain areas serving the highest level of functioning are different in homosexual persons. At this time, these differences do not fit any pattern understandable in terms of what is currently known about prenatal hormonal levels in males and females. Nevertheless, the fact that the differences seem to be in areas of functioning which are known to be affected by hormonal levels (handedness and visuo-spatial ability, for example) would certainly argue that prenatal hormone levels somehow contribute to sexual orientation, at least to some extent or in some people.

Simon LeVay, the neuroscientist who discovered the hypothalamic differences between gay and nongay men, stated: "Homosexuality, like heterosexuality, results at least in part from specific interactions between androgenic sex hormones [testosterone-like hormones] and the brain during development."[21] Dr. LeVay also points out the apparent paradox that a hormonal process during prenatal development which has such a profound effect on sexual behavior seems to have so few other effects in the body. Can the "critical period" of hormonal activity be so precisely timed that a low or high level of testosterone can cause change throughout the brain—but not in the sex organs, muscles, or skeleton? What could cause such a brief burst of hormonal activity? (Not stress during pregnancy, that much seems clear.) Gay men and lesbians differ so slightly from their heterosexual counterparts in every respect aside from their sexual attractions that only the most sophisticated and precise investigations have been able to discover any differences at all between them. Investigation into rare medical conditions indicate that while highly abnormal hormone levels can influence sexual behavior, other effects of abnormal hormone levels, abnormal genitals or body proportions, invariably result in those conditions as well. Clearly, hormone levels are only part of the story.

Hormones are the signals that set in motion patterns of growth— but only if the tissue is designed to receive a particular hormonal signal—and all of these activities are ultimately controlled by genes. It may be that crucial areas of the brain are genetically programmed to respond to testosterone differently in some individuals—the same hormonal "signal" may be "read" differently in different individuals, not because there is a different level of the hormone in the bloodstream but because the tissue may be more or less sensitive to the hormone. What might explain such a difference? In a word: heredity.

NINE

Sexual Genetics

I possess some record of heredity in 32 of my cases [of homosexuality].
Of these, not less than ten assert that they have reason to believe that
other cases of inversion have occurred in their families, and while in
some it is only a strong suspicion, in others there is no doubt whatso-
ever.—Havelock Ellis, *Sexual Inversion*, 1897

Despite these impressive numbers—almost one-third of his subjects
reporting homosexual relatives—Ellis did not "attach great importance to these results." In Germany, Magnus Hirschfeld had noted a
striking family clustering of male homosexuality, reporting that 35
percent of the brothers of his homosexual subjects were also homosexual.[1] Hirschfeld interpreted this data to support his view that homosexuality was a biological phenomenon—not psychologically caused
and certainly not a moral failing. Others, however, interpreted this
data in a very different way.

Genetics was yet to come into its own as a scientific discipline at the
end of the nineteenth century. Although chromosomes had been visu-
alized under the microscope years before and were believed to be
involved in heredity in some way, the mechanisms by which traits were
passed from parents to offspring were poorly understood. The discovery of DNA was half a century away. Modern genetics was only
beginning to develop as a branch of biology, and medicine and the

behavioral sciences remained mired in the outdated speculations of degeneracy theory. Any scientific discussion of hereditary factors in the determination of sexual orientation invariably became an exploration of "neuropathic taint." Alcoholism, insanity, syphilis, "neurasthenia," homosexuality, and even "eccentricity" were seen as expressions of degenerate genetic stock. (The legacy of degeneracy theory remains with us today in that pedophiles, exhibitionists, and other persons with abnormalities of sexual behavior are still sometimes referred to as "degenerates.") The theory proposed that a factor that was an expression of one "degeneracy" in one generation might be the cause of another expression in the next. Alcoholism in one generation might contribute to homosexuality in the next—syphilis might have the same effect. Even masturbation was thought by some to cause a decline in the genetic stock which could manifest itself as neurasthenia or "imbecility" (mental retardation) in the next generation.

The central flaw of degeneracy theory is its reliance on inaccurate inheritance theory (sometimes called Lamarckian theory after the Frenchman who first developed the idea), which holds that *acquired* traits can be transmitted to offspring. Engaging in unhealthy habits such as masturbation or too much alcohol was thought to cause degeneration of the "germ cells" that were passed on to the next generation, resulting in "degenerate conditions" such as mental retardation or homosexuality. It is now known that truly genetic traits are unalterable. Except for direct damage to the DNA molecules in sperm or egg cells caused by agents such as radiation exposure, the genetic material is passed on essentially unchanged from parents to offspring.

Perhaps it is to his credit that Havelock Ellis, who was seeking to promote some measure of understanding and tolerance for homosexuals, downplayed the significance of the family histories of his subjects. This does not mean that he discounted heredity in homosexual orientation. On the contrary, one reason he opposed attempts to "treat" homosexuality by recommending heterosexual marriage to them was to prevent homosexuals from having children. Ellis warned, "In the most successful cases we have simply put into the invert's hands a power of reproduction which it is undesirable he should possess."[2]

Freud, as might be expected, was practically silent on the issue of heredity and sexual orientation. Aside from early, rather vague references to "predispositions" that might be inherited, Freud seemed to have little interest in heredity. (Unlike Ellis, Freud reserved special contempt for degeneracy theory.) Later psychoanalysts discounted genetic influences completely, formulating the development of sexuality completely in psychological terms—free from any biological influences, including heredity.

Alfred Kinsey also downplayed genetic factors in sexual orientation—one of the few instances in which his opinions on sexual behavior coincided with those of the psychoanalysts. The idea of a hereditary predisposition for homosexuality was not consistent with Kinsey's view that sexual orientation was the product of accumulated pleasurable experiences in an individual's early life. Kinsey's main argument against a genetic component to sexual orientation was based, as might be expected, on statistical analysis of his survey data. Kinsey knew that proving any genetic component to homosexual behavior would necessitate proving that the incidence of homosexuality is higher among relatives of homosexuals than in the general population. Persons who share genes would also be expected to share traits—if the traits are genetically based—at a rate higher than in the general population. But since Kinsey's definition of homosexuality was so loose, his numbers for the incidence of homosexuality in the general population are difficult to interpret. In the final analysis, Kinsey believed that homosexual behavior was so common that finding an excess of homosexuality in any group would be impossible.

Twins

As Kinsey's first book was being reviewed (and frequently reviled) in the popular press, the Department of Medical Genetics of the New York State Psychiatric Institute of Columbia University was designing a study to investigate genetic influences on the development of homosexuality in males. Since Magnus Hirschfeld's records of thousands of case histories had been destroyed by the Nazis, there were no large-scale studies that investigated genetic issues in sexual orientation. Dr. Franz Kallmann set about to investigate the issue.

The resulting report, appearing in the British *Journal of Nervous and Mental Disease* in 1952, is remarkable.[3] In the first several paragraphs, Kallmann complains that his subjects were distrustful of his investigators, making inconvenient demands, such as meeting in neutral public places for their interviews, and being uncooperative about discussing their family histories. Kallmann admits later in the paper that his subjects were "still subject to the laws of the State of New York"—alluding to the dire consequences for them if their identities were to be discovered. Smirking contempt for the "clandestine homosexual world" pervades the report. Kallmann acknowledges with "pleasure" the cooperation of the New York State and New York City Departments of Correction and Parole, the work of his field investigators, and even that of his statisticians, but offers not a single word of thanks to the hundred or so men who jeopardized their careers by agreeing to participate in the study—only a disdainful comment: "It has been interesting to confirm that the problems and attitudes of a sexually aberrant group look less wholesome in the twilight of gloomy hiding places than they do from the perspective of . . . a comfortable therapeutic couch."[4] (By contrast, Alfred Kinsey had dedicated his first book to "the 12,000 persons who ha[d] contributed their data.")[5] Kallmann's acknowledgment section also reveals a serious flaw in the study—like Krafft-Ebing's cases in *Psychopathia Sexualis*, most of his subjects came from mental institutions or prisons.

Much of the paper is devoted to an attempt to confirm a previous researcher's bogus theory that gay men have a "defective" Y chromosome and thus have more sisters than brothers in their sibships. (The theory was that most males with a defective Y chromosome should die in utero.) Kallmann's subjects did indeed seem to have slightly more than the expected number of sisters, but analysis revealed that the difference was not statistically significant.

The more interesting part of the study was an analysis of homosexual twins. Kallmann managed to find eighty-five gay men who were twins and was able to interview all but twenty-two of their twin brothers. The results are striking, to say the least.

First, though, a word about twins. Individuals who develop simultaneously during a single human pregnancy are of two types: monozygotic and dizygotic. Monozygotic (also called "identical") twins develop from a single fertilized egg (*mono-*, one; *zygote*, the fertilized egg). After the first division of the fertilized cell, the two new cells separate. Each goes on to develop into a complete individual embryo. Monozygotic twins thus share 100 percent of their genetic material, which accounts for the fact that they are "identical" in appearance. Monozygotic twins are literally genetic "clones." Dizygotic twins result when two ova are simultaneously released from the mother's ovary at ovulation and each is fertilized by a different sperm cell. They share as much genetic material as ordinary brothers or sisters do (hence the label "fraternal twins"); indeed, dizygotic twins may be of two different sexes. Since they develop simultaneously in the uterus, they also share the milieu of the pregnancy: whatever maternal health factors are operating—poor nutrition, infection, drug use—affect both twins equally. The simultaneous occurrence of a trait in each of a set of twins is called "concordance," and twins who share a trait are said to be "concordant" for that trait. Genetic traits would be expected to occur simultaneously more often in monozygotic twins than in dizygotic twins because monozygotic twins are more alike genetically.

In Kallmann's sets of twins, the dizygotic pairs showed an 11.5 percent concordance rate for homosexuality—but the monozygotic sets were reported to show a nearly 100 percent concordance rate. Kallmann's interpretations of these results are a confused mélange of early genetic theory and psychoanalytic speculations such as "only two males who are typical in both the genotypical and the developmental aspects of sexual maturation and personality integration are also apt to be alike in those specific vulnerabilities favoring a trend toward fixation or regression to immature levels of sexuality." Despite the fact that many of Kallmann's conclusions are couched in the murky analytic terminology that characterizes almost all writing on behavioral research of his time, Kallmann's data "weakens the significance of explanations which over-stress . . . factors such as parental incompetence in the etiology of adult homosexuality."[6] Although he did not totally discount the role of upbringing and childhood experiences, Kallmann proposed a significant role for heredity in the development of homosexuality.

One of the problems with the data has already been mentioned: many of the subjects were institutionalized. In addition, Kallmann did not discuss how he decided which twins were monozygotic and which were dizygotic—a task more difficult than one might think. The main criticism of the study at the time it was published, however, was that Kallmann's twins grew up together and therefore were subject to the same rearing practices. It was argued that since the twins shared their environment as well as their genes, the study did not support a genetic factor for homosexuality. To argue that genetic endowment couldn't possibly explain a twin series with 100 percent concordance rate might seem absurd today; nevertheless, Kallmann's study was rejected out of hand by contemporaries. As recently as 1993 his 100 percent concordance was dismissed as "an artifact,"[7] illustrating the ability of entrenched theory to prevail over experimental data regardless of how compelling the data appear.

Although cases of homosexual twins appeared sporadically in ensuing years, it would be almost three decades before another large-scale study of homosexuality in twins would be attempted. In 1991, more than a hundred male twin pairs were analyzed by J. Michael Bailey of Northwestern University and Richard Pillard of the Boston University School of Medicine.[8] Two years later, a similar study of female twin pairs was published.[9] The twins were recruited by advertisements in gay community publications in the midwestern and southwestern United States; gay or bisexual individuals over the age of eighteen who had twins or adoptive siblings were asked to contact the researchers. Bailey and Pillard carefully analyzed the sexual orientation of the volunteers and were able to interview in person most of the other twins and the adoptive brothers and sisters.

The results of these two studies strongly suggested that genetic factors operate in the development of sexual orientation. In the men, the monozygotic twins had a 50 percent concordance rate for homosexuality, and the dizygotic twins had a 24 percent concordance rate. The adoptive brothers had a 19 percent concordance rate. In the female study 48 percent of the monozygotic pairs were concordant for homosexuality, as were 16 percent of the dizygotic pairs and 6 percent of the pairs of adoptive sisters. Summarizing the concordance rates for homosexuality, we obtain the following:

	MONOZYGOTIC TWINS	DIZYGOTIC TWINS	ADOPTIVE SIBLINGS
Males	50%	24%	19%
Females	48%	16%	6%

The concordance rates for sexual orientation follow the pattern that would be expected for a genetic trait: the twins who were more alike genetically (the monozygotic pairs) had a higher concordance rate than the twins who were not as similar (the dizygotic pairs and adoptive siblings).

One piece of data from the male study seems rather odd. The concordance rate for the adoptive brothers was 19 percent, almost as high as that for the dizygotic twins. Adoptive brothers are genetic "strangers"; they should have no more in common genetically than two men picked at random from the general population. Why do these "strangers" have almost as high a concordance rate as the dizygotic twins? The authors noticed a difference in the willingness of different groups of gay men volunteering for the study to allow the researchers to contact their brothers. Gay men whose brothers were twins were willing to have their brothers contacted regardless of whether their twin was gay or heterosexual; but the gay men whose brothers were adoptive were often reluctant to have their brother contacted if he was not gay. Bailey and Pillard reasoned that if gay men were reluctant to have a nongay adoptive brother contacted for research, then gay men with nongay adoptive brothers had probably been less likely to volunteer for the study in the first place. This pattern would have resulted in an enriched sample among the adoptive brother pairs—enriched with concordant pairs, thus having a higher concordance rate among adoptive brothers than is really accurate.

By doing their research on twins, Bailey and Pillard avoided the pitfall that Kinsey had predicted would make study of the heredity of sexual orientation impossible—the need for knowledge of the incidence rate of homosexuality in the general population. This study compares rates of homosexuality in groups with differing degrees of relatedness: genetically identical (the monozygotic pairs), genetically similar (the dizygotic pairs), and genetically unrelated (the adoptive siblings). As would be expected if heredity plays a significant role in the development of sexual orientation, the more closely related the individuals, the higher the concordance rate.

As carefully designed as these studies were, they have been harshly criticized. It has been pointed out that since the subjects were recruited through gay community publications, the group studied was not representative of all homosexuals but only of those who read, as the authors of one critical article put it, "homosexually oriented periodicals."[10] This view would propose that gay men and lesbians who read gay community newspapers are a unique group, perhaps fundamentally different in their development from those who do not. The other criticism is that it may be the differing treatment of sets of identical twins and fraternal twins which accounts for the difference in their concordance rates. The ghostly voice of Sigmund Freud can be heard once more in the pronouncement of one critic who stated, "The problem is more important in homosexuality . . . because [identical] twins grow up with mirror images of themselves that can magnify their so-called narcissism." This writer argued that the more similar appearance of monozygotic twins somehow leads the parents of such twins to treat them more alike than fraternal twins would be treated.[11] This argument would propose that the higher concordance rates for monozygotic twins are due, not to identical genes, but rather to the fact that identical twins grow up in more similar rearing environments than fraternal twins—another example of how a peculiar possibility can still be used to dismiss research results even in major scientific publications when the topic is homosexuality.

Several more large-scale studies (involving thousands of pairs of twins) completed in the mid-1990s have confirmed the results of these earlier studies. There is now little doubt that sexual orientation is substantially influenced by hereditary factors in both males and females.[12]

Probing the Double Helix

In 1951, the elucidation of the structure of deoxyribonucleic acid, better known as DNA, brought the science of genetics into the modern biochemical age. Scientists had peered through microscopes for more than a century at tiny wormlike structures that mysteriously appeared inside cells preparing to divide and then just as mysteriously disappeared. Although they were certain that these structures, called chromosomes, contained information that was transmitted from parents to offspring, early geneticists remained ignorant of the means by which the information was coded, stored, and replicated. Unraveling the mystery of the structure of DNA revealed an astonishingly simple and elegant mechanism at work.

DNA consists of two long chains of linked molecules (called nucleotides) arranged in a spiral structure called a double helix. The links in each chain are of just four types of nucleotides, and it is the sequence of nucleotides which encodes the genetic information. Just as any amount of written information from "SOS" to the text of *War and Peace* can be translated into Morse code using only dots and dashes, all the genetic information, for blue eyes or brown, straight hair or curly, male or female, is contained on the DNA molecules using the four symbols of the genetic code. The double helix structure makes copies of itself by opening along its length like a zipper unzipping, each half acting as a template for a new and identical daughter molecule. The chromosomes appearing during cell division are DNA molecules coiled and packaged for easy and safe distribution to two new cells.

DNA determines the structures of the body by coding for the manufacture of proteins such as myosin (muscle protein), hemoglobin (the oxygen-carrying protein of red blood cells), and collagen (the structural protein of skin and cartilage). Proteins called enzymes direct the manufacture of nonprotein substances that make up the structure of the body (bones from calcium salts, for example) or are responsible for other aspects of bodily functioning (the secretion of stomach acid, for example). Many hormones are proteins (like insulin), and even hormones that are not proteins (like testosterone, estrogen, and the other steroid hormones) are manufactured by protein enzymes. Proteins like nerve-growth factors (NGFs) are present only briefly during development to signal the growth of certain cells and the development of particular structures; when their work is done, they disappear. The complex structure of the body is built from or manufactured by proteins; its functioning is controlled by proteins or by substances manufactured by proteins—and the structure of all these proteins is determined by the genetic signals encoded on the DNA molecule. Although chromosomal DNA is not the only informational system operative in heredity, it is by far the most important.

In addition to the sections of DNA which code for proteins (structural genes), other sections control the *timing* of gene activity (regulatory genes), turning the structural genes on and off at critical times. (Some forms of cancer are thought to result from a malfunction of genes that turn on growth processes inappropriately.) Although the DNA molecule contains almost all the information needed for the development and biological functioning of the body in a code that is, in fact, now readable, we are a long way from being able to read the DNA molecule.

Until quite recently however, "reading" DNA was possible only after it had been randomly chopped up into short lengths. Imagine for a moment that ten New York City phone books have been put through a shredding machine—several times—so that the information they contained is now scattered among millions of tiny bits of paper each containing only a few letters and numbers. Only with a monumental amount of matching and categorization of the bits would it eventually be possible to reconstruct the information. Identifying genes was a similarly daunting endeavor—until the discovery of restriction endonucleases. These chemical probes are capable of clipping out sections

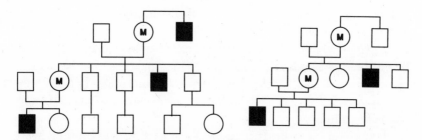

Two family pedigrees from the initial study of the inheritance of male homo-sexuality by Dean Hamer and his colleagues ("A Linkage between DNA Markers on the X Chromosome and Male Sexual Orientation," *Science* 261 [July 16, 1993]: 321–27). These family trees show gay men (*solid squares*) whose mothers (*open circles marked with an M*) have gay brothers. In these families, homosexuality was passed through the mother's X chromosome.

of DNA at specific sites. Though still quite challenging, the task of reassembly has been substantially simplified with these tools. (The discovery of restriction enzymes was such a tremendous breakthrough in genetics that it earned the codiscoverers, Daniel Nathans and Ham-ilton Smith of the Johns Hopkins School of Medicine, the Nobel Prize for Medicine in 1978.) Many genes have now been located on particular chromosomes, and many more "markers" have been found. In 1993, a group of geneticists headed by Dean Hamer at the National Institutes of Health who had been using these new techniques to probe the DNA molecule published a paper in the journal *Science* which linked male homosexuality in some families to a particular region of a particular chromosome.[13]

Like previous investigators, Hamer and his colleagues had first looked at the family histories of homosexuals and had found that the family tree of a gay person frequently revealed other gays in the family. In looking at the families of gay men, they found that 13.5 percent of the gay subjects they had recruited for the study had a gay brother, and these men also frequently had a gay uncle or cousin on the mother's side (about 7.5 percent had a gay maternal uncle or maternal cousin). Although not all the family trees showed this pattern, in several fam-ilies the inheritance of male homosexuality through the mother's side of the family across several generations was strikingly apparent.

This unmistakable pattern tremendously narrowed the search for the location of a gene—it had to be on the X chromosome. Men always get their X chromosome from their mother; so if a trait is always inherited through their mother, the chromosomal gene involved must be on the X chromosome. (Remember that males have an X and a Y chromosome, while females have two X chromosomes. It is not unusual for an X-linked gene to be "silent" in a female who passes it on to male offspring.)

Hamer and his colleagues found forty pairs of gay brothers who they thought had a good chance of sharing an X chromosome gene—gay brothers whose family did not show inheritance of homosexuality through the father and who had no more than one lesbian relative were studied, eliminating families in which other types of transmission of the trait might be operating. When the DNA markers on the X chromosomes of these brothers were examined, it was found that thirty-three of the forty pairs shared markers at the tip of the long arm of the X chromosome in an area called Xq28. Statistical analysis indicated that the sharing of so many markers could not be explained by chance alone. The results were offered as evidence that in some men, a gene or genes on one end of the X chromosome are strongly linked to homosexuality.

In a later study of a different sample of thirty-two pairs of gay brothers, Hamer and his colleagues again found that a significant majority of the gay brothers shared the Xq28 marker (twenty-three out of thirty-two).[14] In this paper, Hamer also reported on eleven families in which a pair of gay brothers had another brother who was not gay. In nine out of eleven families, the heterosexual brother did *not* have the Xq28 markers that his gay brothers shared. (The study also looked at families with two lesbian sisters and found that there was no correlation between Xq28 and lesbianism. This is consistent with other studies that have failed to demonstrate any genetic link between male and female homosexuality.)

What might such a gene code for? Since so much other evidence for biological factors in sexual orientation involves prenatal hormones, the testosterone receptor was a likely candidate. Several medical conditions have been found to be due to particular defects in this gene. Androgen insensitivity syndrome, the condition in which XY individuals develop with female anatomy, is caused by a mutation at one end of the gene for the testosterone receptor. When the gene for the testosterone receptor was analyzed in the gay brothers, however, it turned out that there was nothing unique about the gene for the testosterone receptor in these men.[15] In contrast to the striking concordance of markers at Xq28, the testosterone receptor genes showed random variations between the brothers as well as between the groups of gay men and nongay men.

Androgen insensitivity syndrome isn't the only medical disorder that is caused by a defect in the gene for the testosterone receptor. Spinal bulbar muscular atrophy (SBMA), a degenerative neurological condition characterized by progressive degeneration of the nerve cells controlling muscular movements, is also caused by a defect in a portion of the gene for the testosterone receptor. The point here is that genes may have functions that at first seem far afield from what is expected— why does a testosterone receptor defect cause a degeneration of nerve cells of the muscular system? Genes may have different functions during different stages of development. Since there is so much evidence that the hormonal events that seem to be correlated with homosexuality occur only briefly during the earliest stages of development of the brain, the identification of the function of the Xq28 gene will be a daunting task.

In one very important way, though, the results of the genetic studies mirror some of the conclusions from the hormonal studies, studies of handedness and psychological testing, and other biological correlates of homosexuality. Heredity only partially accounts for the development of sexual orientation. Although about 50 percent of identical twins showed concordance for homosexuality in the Bailey studies, 50 percent did not. The sharing of identical genes does not predict identical outcome in the development of sexual orientation. In one of the families Hamer and his colleagues studied, four brothers shared the Xq28 markers, but two of them were gay and the other two were not. Although a number of the families studied by Hamer and his colleagues showed a genetic influence apparently passed down through the X chromosome, not all the families with gay brothers showed this pattern of inheritance. This would suggest that genes other than the Xq28 might be involved in male homosexuality.

These findings would seem to indicate that even the fullest possible understanding of the biological underpinnings of sexual orientation will tell only a portion of the story of homosexuality. All the work on hormones, handedness, and genes leaves out one very important element, which for lack of a better word might be called the human element. In Part Three, "Sexual Identities," we will leave behind molecules and pedigrees and start to look at people and their experiences. First, however, in the next chapter, I'll try to pull all the facts of this part of the book together and address that nagging debate over "nature versus nurture."

TEN

Nature *and* Nurture

New theories of the workings of the brain and of the relationship between the brain and the "mind" indicate that dichotomies such as "nature versus nurture" and "psychological versus biological" do not make very much sense when complex human behaviors are considered. In this chapter I hope to persuade you that to ask "nature or nurture" questions about homosexuality doesn't make sense, either. Human sexuality, like our capacity for language and the complex set of capacities we call "intelligence," can *only* be understood as arising from a complex interplay of nature *and* nurture, psychology *and* biology, genes *and* environment.

The Self-Wiring Brain

In the rat, there are as many genes governing the development of the brain as there are for all the other organs and tissues combined.[1] Even this immense amount of genetic material cannot possibly code for all the connections between all the neurons in the brain. In the human brain there are eleven billion neurons, and each neuron may make contact with and transmit signals to up to fifty thousand other neurons. The number of possible connections between neurons is incomprehensibly large, a hyperastronomical number on the order of the number of molecules in the universe. The information contained in an individual's DNA could not possibly code for these connections except in a very general way. Genes are now thought to code only for *general* patterns of connections; the *specific* patterns come later. As biologist Robert Wesson puts it, "The genome [all the genetic material in an organism] is not a blueprint . . . but a set of instructions."[2] The brain "wires" itself—largely *after* birth—in response to information from the environment.

One still occasionally hears the functioning of the brain and nervous system compared to that of a computer. This is a vast oversimplification. The brain is not like a computer with eleven billion switches; it is more like a network of eleven billion computers, each one capable of being individually programmed. Lower-level neurons are narrowly tuned to receive specific kinds of information: the neurons in the retina of the eye respond to a certain wavelength of light at a certain position in the visual field; auditory cells in the ear respond to sound of a certain frequency. Higher-level neurons receive these sets of signals, perform sorting operations, and assemble information. One set of neurons compares information with another set, and complex feedback loops allow the interaction of many different kinds of information from different areas of the brain. Networks of neurons become functionally linked such that information from one resonates with and calls up action from another. The development of these networks and their linkage to one another come about through interaction with information from outside the organism—by a process we usually call "learning."

In the 1940s, scientists discovered the brain's "self-wiring" by studying human infants who could not learn to see. Before the advent of antibiotics, infants with certain infections were born with a clouding of the clear parts of the eye. This clouding prevented their retina from receiving a focused image, and these children, though able to distinguish light from dark, were for all practical purposes blind. When new surgical techniques were developed making it possible to replace the cloudy parts with normal tissue, it was discovered that these individuals still could not "see," even though their eyes now functioned normally. It became apparent that the areas of the brain which processed the signals from the eyes were not doing their job properly. The brain could not make use of the information coming from the now normal eyes. Experiments with animals soon revealed the problem: the visual system of the newborn's brain needs visual input from the eyes during the first several weeks of life in order to organize itself. If the signals from the eyes are not properly transmitted during this critical period, this capacity for self-assembly is lost forever. The visual system is preprogrammed to receive information from the environment and to organize itself in response to that information. As one examines animals of increasing complexity, the length of time it takes for this to occur becomes longer. The process goes on for the first three months of a cat's life, the first year of a monkey's, and the first two years of a human's. This is the now familiar concept of the "critical period." As we've seen, the brain exhibits a critical period response to certain hormonal events. The big question before us now is, Does as complex a phenomenon as homosexuality arise from similar neurological events, or are there other influences? To try to answer this question, let's turn for a moment to another complex phenomenon that is uniquely human: language.

Sexual orientation has been compared to native language—an individual has only one native language per lifetime. He or she can learn other languages, even speak them fluently and effortlessly—but a second language will never be spoken with the ease and "naturalness" of one's native tongue. Like sexual orientation, native language seems "embedded" in the brain at a certain point and not subject to change. Is this comparison a valid one?

Only humans possess true language abilities. Although with an enormous amount of training, chimps can learn to associate hand signals with various objects, they lack true language ability. A chimp might be capable of being trained to "say" something like "Give me the banana," but even something marginally more complicated, such as "I liked the banana that you gave me yesterday," is completely beyond the creature's capacity. Humans, on the other hand, have a brain that is ready within about a year of birth to begin the process of acquiring language—any language. Human children learn English as easily as they learn Italian or Chinese or Masai. The human brain has an inborn language capacity that is stimulated by exposure to *any* language, from Armenian to Zoque.

The process of language acquisition in humans also exhibits the critical period phenomenon. Immigrants to a new country will speak the language of their new home with more or less of an accent depending on the age at which they learn their new language. The older the age at which the second language is learned, the more difficult it will be to speak without an accent. Humans reach a "point of no return" at about age six, when the native language is set. Although individuals can learn additional new languages beyond this age, they do so by a different kind of learning. A two-year-old placed in an environment in which a new language is spoken will learn to speak it without any special effort or direction—a twenty-year-old will not, as anyone taking up a new language in college knows full well. If language areas of the brain are damaged, the extent to which individuals will recover language ability depends primarily on their age. Children who suffer brain damage recover substantial language skills, whereas injured teenagers remain more severely impaired. Adult stroke victims may remain permanently aphasic (without any language capacity at all).

How is language encoded in the brain? Several types of evidence suggest that language capacity is embedded in the structure and biology of the human brain. There is an anatomy of language—certain brain areas are necessary for various language functions. In addition, language follows other biological rules: a critical period phenomenon is observed, and certain universal grammatical elements of all human languages suggest that the same organizational structure underlies all of them.

Some biologists believe that the development of the human capacity for language (among other capacities) came about during evolution as a result of a process called *neoteny*. Neoteny is a developmental phenomenon in which the maturation of certain organ systems is delayed. As one moves up the evolutionary scale, it is apparent that the period of time needed for maturation from newborn to adult becomes longer and longer. Puppies and kittens are "babies" for a longer time after birth than are newborn mice. Baby chimps must be cared for by their mothers for still longer, and human infants remain helpless for an even longer period of time. Much of this increase in maturation time is needed for the maturation of the brain.

Examination of a behavior pattern common among many different animals will illustrate the relationship between neoteny and learning. Many animals have a "hunting instinct" that is varyingly capable of elaboration and development through learning processes. The "hunting" behavior of fish and frogs, basically lunging open-mouthed at just about anything that moves, is crude and unsophisticated. Mother fish don't need to teach this skill to their fry—who seem to be "prewired" for the behavior. The stealth and pursuit behaviors of lions and panthers, on the other hand, involve significant learning. Some behaviors are learned from adults, and some through trial and error and "play" behavior. It is thought that "playfulness" in immature animals is linked to learning and intelligence. Animal species who are the most adventuresome and curious as youngsters are also the most intelligent—as anyone knows who has observed the differences in playfulness between puppies or kittens and, say, baby mice.

To be capable of more complex behavior, especially learned behavior, the brain *must* be more immature at birth and develop over a longer period of time. The "hard-wired" brain of lower animals is not capable of flexible adaptation to a changing environment because a "hard-wired" brain cannot learn. As stated above, the details of brain organization cannot possibly be encoded in the genes. Complex capacities such as language—not to mention mental processes like mathematics, musical composition, or theology—are possible only if brain development is delayed for a fairly long period after birth and thus relatively free to organize itself and be responsive to a wide variety of types of information from the environment. This open-ended capacity for development may be what separates us from lower animals. Animals have instincts that help them survive in their environment; only humans have the ability to learn from the environment and fit themselves to it—or it to them.

What is the biology of this learning process? Modern theories of mental functioning emphasize that learning occurs through the development of networks of neurons. Terms such as *neuronal group selection*, *cortical networks*, and *neural nets* all refer to aspects of this theory. Vastly oversimplified, it states that learning occurs as complex patterns of linkage develop between neurons.

The brain is thought to start out with a simple, symmetrical neural architecture. As information is received from the environment, a gradual strengthening of connections between some neurons and the weakening of connections between others give rise to "networks" with specific functions in the brain. Before learning, neurons are all loosely functionally connected. A symmetrical network exists (as shown on the next page).

As learning occurs, connections are strengthened between some cells and weakened between others. Patterns and pathways develop as some neurons become functionally linked. With further experience and learning, the anatomy of the circuit begins to change even further, and more complex patterns develop. These changes of circuitry proba-

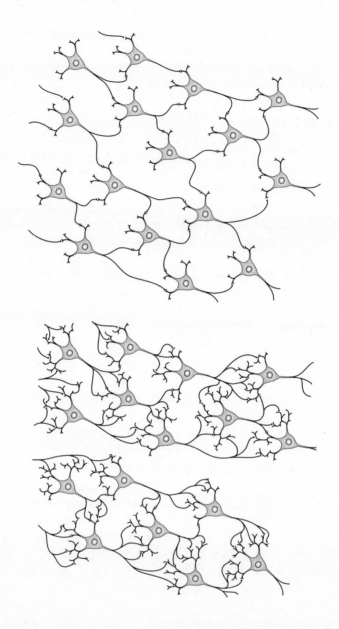

Top, A developing neural network, showing similar connections between similar cells. *Bottom*, A later network, showing increased and more complex linkages between some cells and loss of linkages between others. Definite pathways have now developed which will be permanent.

bly involve chemical changes within the neurons as well as structural changes. Neurons sprout new filaments and establish new connections with neighboring neurons. Ever more complex patterns and networks within networks develop as experiences continue to stimulate learning.

This conceptualization of the learning process in the brain will make perfect sense to anyone who has learned to play a musical instrument. A new piano student must laboriously decipher the meaning of the notes and fingerings on a written page of music and then *consciously* "translate" them into specific piano keys that are played with specific fingers. With more practice the process becomes easier, and less conscious thought is required. Eventually the visual image of the written music is effortlessly and "automatically" translated into finger movements on the keyboard. What were once individual mental steps— reading the music, translating the notes into their names ("middle C," "B flat," and so forth), finding the named keys on the keyboard, and playing the keys with the correct fingers—are now seamlessly linked into a single process. Learning to speak, to read, to use a typewriter, to throw a baseball, to drive a car—all learning seems to operate the same way.

To what extent can these connections be rearranged and the learning process reversed? The process of "forgetting" may result from gradual unlinking within a network owing to low activity of the connections. This seems to vary according to the behavior in question. Some behaviors, however, seem to be *permanently* imprinted: one doesn't forget how to walk. Some behaviors become deeply embedded in the structure of the brain—native language is a good example. A person can learn to speak and even to think in a new language, but each individual has only one native language. Learning new languages depends, at least at first, on a translation process from the new language into the primary one. Once one's native language is established, only brain injury can abolish it.

Value Centers

Although containing much less "hard wiring" than those of simpler animals, the human brain is not, as earlier philosophers sometimes called it, a "tabula rasa"—a blank slate. Several findings indicate that at least some brain "circuitry" is "hard wired," even in humans. There are

some circuits that operate with only a minimal need for learning processes. There is, for example, a circuitry for fear. It includes the brain,
the adrenal glands (which secrete the "fight or flight" hormone, adren-
aline), and the vagus nerve (which exerts nervous control over heart
rate and blood pressure). Although some degree of learning can aug-
ment or suppress these responses, a limitation on the range of the
response seems to be imposed on the system, perhaps genetically.
These limits have been called "value centers."[3] It is reasonable to
suppose that the most important value centers have to do with self-
preservation and the preservation of the species. A "maternal instinct"
is present in practically every species of bird and mammal and seems to
rely little on learning processes. Most female animals do not need to
learn how to take care of their young. The brain circuitry is already in
place and is probably activated by hormonal changes that occur during
pregnancy. In most species, male animals ferociously compete with
each other for reproductive privileges. Their energies are devoted to
self-preservation and to copulation with the greatest possible number
of females. Their value centers are different from the females' but are
just as powerful. A genetic basis for value centers makes perfect sense
in classic evolutionary theory—behaviors will be perpetuated during
evolution and encoded in the genes that maximize the number of
offspring.

In humans, however, the brain and nervous system have developed
capacities that seem to have little to do with increasing reproductive
success. Intelligence is a good example; it has never been demonstrated
that higher intelligence increases reproductive success in humans.[4]
Humans are much more intelligent than they need to be to maximize
reproduction. Altruism, the sacrifice of one's own comfort or available
resources in order to benefit others, is an almost uniquely human trait.
It seems to violate one of the basic tenets of classical evolutionary
theory: survival of the fittest and extinction of the weak. Where have
these sorts of behaviors come from?

In humans, complex interpersonal bondings take place which have
absolutely no counterpart in the animal world. Not only altruism but
family loyalty, spousal devotion, friendship, patriotism, and even spiritual dedication are but a few of the kinds of bondings which humans
are capable of forming. It would seem that in the human animal a
capacity for bonding exists which, though it perhaps builds on a reproductive value center, has far more symbolic aims than the propaga-

tion of the species. While animals can at most form groups of individuals loosely organized into packs or troops, humans have formed societies and cultures. Only humans are capable of becoming passionate about ideas.

It is reasonable to suppose that value centers for behavior have gradually become more and more attenuated in humans. Intelligence increases not only with size of the brain but also with the learning capacity allowed by its architecture. If intelligence is the capacity for learning, it is also the absence of instinct. As biologist Robert Wesson has stated, "For an animal to become more intelligent means to enlarge the open-ended capability at the expense of semi-hardwiring."[5]

A Sexual Theory

The complete story of the biological correlates of sexual orientation is far from complete, but it is possible to assemble existing scientific data into a theory that fits the known facts.

Prenatal hormonal levels determine much of what is typical male and typical female behavior in animals—all the experimentation with hormonally treated rats makes this much clear. In humans, the study of rare medical conditions indicates that prenatal hormonal events also influence human behaviors. The data on girls with congenital adrenal hyperplasia who tended to be "tomboys" point in this direction, as do other data discussed in previous chapters.

Studies of brain anatomy, of differences in rates of right-handedness versus left-handedness, and of differential performances on psychological tests indicate that the brain organization of gay men and lesbians is different from their heterosexual peers—different in characteristics that have been shown in animals to also be affected by prenatal hormone levels. (Remember the testosterone-treated female rats who had better navigational ability than nontreated females?)

Compared with other animals, the behavioral differences between human males and human females are small. It is thought that this is because the human brain is not affected by testosterone during development nearly as much as the brains of other animals. The levels of male hormones normally secreted during prenatal development are not high enough to produce the fullest possible expression of male behavior in human males.[6] Thus, "maleness" and "femaleness" in the male and female human brain, while measurably different across large groups, overlap considerably. Decreased male aggressiveness may be the most significant result of this downward modulation of neural "maleness," a modulation that may allow for increased involvement of the male in parenting as well as the male-male and nonsexual male-female cooperation necessary for the development of complex societies and culture.

Humans show a wide variety of intense bonding behaviors. Some, like "falling in love," seem understandable as an expression of a reproductive value center, but others, like patriotism, do not. In humans, the connection between interpersonal attachment and reproduction seems much looser and subject to variability—perhaps also a result of the overlap between male and female neural organization. There is less in the way of "hard wiring" in the human brain compared with the brains of lower animals. Perhaps, as discussed above, this is a prerequisite for our intelligence and enormous capacity for learning. It is not too great a theoretical leap to imagine that genetic variations in the hormonal control of brain development result, in some individuals, in an even greater "loosening" of the link between reproductive behavior and emotional attachment. These individuals would have the same capacity (and need) for emotional attachment but would be less "hard wired" for attachment to members of the opposite sex than their peers—more open ended in their capacity to "fall in love." The mysterious childhood psychological and developmental cues that lead to sexual attraction can steer them toward sexual attraction to their own gender—or to both genders—because they are less predetermined in their orientation toward reproductive partners.

Perhaps individuals more likely to develop homosexual orientation are those who are less "hard wired" for reproduction than their peers. This line of reasoning is also consistent with the evidence that sexual orientation is under *some* genetic control but that other factors must be operating as well. Remember that 50 percent of the gay twins studied by Bailey and Pillard had a nongay identical twin brother.

Evidence from the neurobiology of development and learning explains why sexual orientation does not appear to be subject to change. Some behaviors, even behaviors acquired exclusively through learning, such as language, become embedded in the structure of the nervous system as they develop. By puberty, the brain has lost most of its capacity to undergo fundamental change. If sexual orientation is also one of these embedded behavioral characteristics, it should be no more possible to change one's sexual orientation than it would be to change one's native language—an idea that Havelock Ellis and Sigmund Freud and millions of gay men and lesbians would find quite consistent with their experiences.

New findings in the study of behavior indicate that it is impossible to separate "nature" from "nurture," or "psychological" processes from "biological" processes. Some human experiences can be understood as more biological than psychological—hunger and pain, for example. But even these very biological experiences can be highly influenced by the psychic: Hindu mystics walk on hot coals without feeling pain during states of religious ecstasy.

Other experiences seem more exclusively of "mind" rather than of "brain"—philosophy and poetry, for example. Some human experiences seem embedded in our brain but called into action only by experience and learning—like our capacity for language. But in no aspect of human behavior are our biological and psychological selves so melded and intertwined as in our sexuality.

Sexual orientation seems to follow too many biological "rules" for homosexuality to be nothing but a social "construction." Critical periods, hormonal effects, differences in brain structure and functioning all indicate that there is a biology of sexual orientation. But as Kinsey discovered, individuals cannot be divided into "sheep and goats." And orientation toward one or the other or both genders can occur in many different proportions. Unique life experiences interact with unique biological potentials to produce each individual's unique sexuality.

The complexities of these interactions and the infinite variations of human experiences also explain why no one has ever been able to find a "cause" for homosexuality. Neither Gunter Dörner's theories about hormones nor psychoanalytic theories about cold, distant fathers and overinvolved mothers have been borne out by research.[7] Homosexuality, like most other uniquely human experiences, is too complex to be explained except in human terms. If our most human quality is our enormous diversity of capacities and capabilities, especially in our relationships with each other, it should not be at all surprising that in some of us, the capacity for love becomes oriented toward members of the same sex.

PART III

Sexual Identities

We will now leave behind hormones and neurons and molecules and talk about people. As we have seen, homosexuality is not something that can be measured in a laboratory or seen under a microscope or on an MRI scan. Although biological and chemical correlates of sexual orientation have been discovered (and more seem to get discovered all the time), it is impossible to understand homosexuality without getting to know individuals and hearing their stories. We've already heard several, such as those of Anne Lister, Karl Ulrichs, and John Addington Symonds. In this part of the book, we'll take a closer look at the process by which individuals come to think of themselves as homosexual. Although this process is unique to each individual, most people who come to identify themselves as homosexual share many experiences and milestones on the way to a gay or lesbian identity; understanding these experiences provides another perspective on homosexuality.

Although some social scientists still insist that homosexuality is fiendishly difficult to study because it is impossible to define, most individuals—most adults at least—seem to have little difficulty deciding whether they are homosexual. In the genetic study by Dean Hamer discussed in Chapter 9, more than 90 percent of the men studied identified themselves on the Kinsey scale as either 0 or 1 (exclusively or nearly exclusively heterosexual) or as 5 or 6 (exclusively or nearly exclusively homosexual). When the researchers looked only at sexual fantasy and attraction, the two groups moved even further apart, more than 95 percent of the subjects being at one end or the other of the scale. Some research indicates that sexual orientation in women is more diffuse, with more women reporting sexual responsiveness to either sex—but the large majority of women still identify themselves as either lesbian or heterosexual.

Despite the easy certainty about sexual orientation which most adults report, only a moment's thought tells us that young children have no concept of sexual orientation and would simply be bewildered by the question "Are you homosexual?" What happens between childhood and adulthood in an individual that makes him or her come to identify himself or herself as having a sexual orientation? What is the process by which people come to identify themselves as homosexual—and can it tell us something about the phenomenon of sexual orientation? In the next two chapters I will try to answer these questions one at a time.

In the last chapter of Part Three, we will explore the still perplexing issue of bisexuality, a sexual identity that has yet to be understood nearly as well as homosexuality, as well as some identities and behaviors that have come to be called transgender phenomena: transsexualism and transvestism.

ELEVEN

Homosexual Identity Development

The process by which people in our society come to identify themselves as homosexual persons is surprisingly consistent from one person to the next. Several large-scale studies have interviewed thousands of gay men and lesbians, and several scientists have written extensively on the process that has come to be called "homosexual identity development."

Identity formation can be simplified substantially if it is thought of as a process of self-labeling—a person recognizing that a particular label applies to himself or herself. Although many people try to distance themselves from the idea of labeling other people, humans seem to have an inordinate interest in categorizing themselves. One need only pick up an issue or two of the various popular magazines about psychology to find any number of "quizzes" that purport to provide readers with profound insights about themselves, often by helping them decide whether they fit into this category or that one. People check off answers to questions about what they do at parties or what kind of pet they have or even what colors appeal to them to find out whether they are "intuitive" or "analytic," "emotional" or "rational," and then wonder how to put this knowledge to some practical use. Who has eaten in a Chinese restaurant in this country and not used a "Chinese Zodiac" on the menu to find out his or her "compatibilities" as derived from the year of his or her birth? Since there have been various labels for a person's sexual orientation for about a thousand years now, it should come as no surprise that self-labeling in such a profoundly important area as our sexual lives is, as historian John Boswell puts it, "urgent, intuitive and profoundly important."[1]

The first step in this process is learning the labels and understanding the categories. In sexual orientation identity formation, it's fairly clear that the first step happens before the second—children learn the labels for sexual orientation several years before they are capable of understanding the concept of sexual orientation. It's unfortunate that the labels children learn first are usually terms of derision. Elementary school children can be heard using words like *sissy*, *tomboy*, and even *queer* and *faggot* as terms of contempt for each other years before they have mature sexual feelings or become familiar with concepts of sexual orientation.

Although children use the labels of sexual orientation, they use them differently than adults do. A visit to any schoolyard will confirm that children left to their own devices will segregate during play along lines of gender. In a playground full of children under the age of ten or so, boys will be observed to play with boys and girls with girls. Research has confirmed that this is true across many cultures. It has also been shown that the kind of play children usually engage in depends on their gender. We've already touched on "rough and tumble play" in children: boys tend to be more active and rowdy. Choice of toys differs as well: when given choices, boys tend to pick "boy" toys (toy trucks, for example). Girls will play with either dolls or "boy" toys, but they are more likely to show nurturing behaviors (playing with dolls, for example) in their play than boys. Although young children do not normally show sexual behaviors, many of their behaviors can be classified along gender lines. Thus, play among young children is gender differentiated.

Although they are ignorant of mature concepts of sexual orientation, children are exquisitely sensitive to gender roles at a very young age, and children who do not conform to expectations of gender-differentiated behavior are frequently taunted and ridiculed. Often the epithets applied to homosexuals are used as the verbal weapons. During childhood, then, an association begins to develop between words like *sissy* and *queer* and particular behaviors: gender-nonconforming behaviors. Children also begin to associate these words with being different and unwanted.

When adult homosexuals are interviewed, many (but not all) report that they felt "different" from other children when they were young. Frequently, when questioned more closely, it turns out that this sense of "differentness" came from the fact that they had play interests of the opposite gender during childhood. Boys may find they are less interested in sports than their peers and prefer solitary activities such as reading and music; girls may find that they are more independent or athletic than other girls. All of this occurs completely outside the realm of sexuality at this age, in what might be called the social world of the child, the world of friends and games and school. Richard Isay, a psychiatrist who has written extensively on psychotherapy with gay men, states: "Every gay man I have seen reports that beginning at age 3 or 4 he experienced that he was 'different' from his peers. This feeling is described as having been more sensitive, crying more easily, having his feelings hurt more readily, having aesthetic interests, and being less aggressive than others of his age. Such differences make children feel like outsiders in relation to peers and often to family as well."[2] Many now believe that such a childhood pattern of interests and socialization represents a nonerotic expression of developing homosexuality.

As with just about all the research on homosexuality, there are many exceptions to these findings; the differences between recalled play patterns in homosexual and nonhomosexual persons are not universal. Some persons who as adults consider themselves heterosexual recall also feeling "different" from same-sex peers and engaging in gender-nonconforming play—and some adults who identify themselves as homosexual do not recall these feelings or behaviors. But the pattern is quite striking: in one study, 72 percent of gay men reported feeling "somewhat or very different" from same-sex peers, whereas only 39 percent of a control group of heterosexual men reported similar feelings.[3] (The term *marginalization* has been used to capture the idea of being not quite part of the group.)

Richard Troiden, a social scientist who has written extensively on the identity formation process for homosexuals, has come to label these early experiences of "differentness" as the "sensitization stage" of homosexual identity development, which occurs between the ages of six and twelve.[4] He uses the term *prehomosexual* to emphasize that these children do not usually think of themselves as sexually different and that the term *homosexual* usually holds no significance for them. These children assume that they will grow up to be mommies and daddies just like their parents—that is, heterosexual.

These children are "sensitized" to two things during these years: to a feeling of being different from their same-sex peers, and also to a set of labels and attitudes. The labels may include *homosexual* and *gay* or *lesbian* but also *queer, faggot, dyke,* and so forth. The attitudes are often contempt and aversion, even disgust. Our society's antihomosexual bias is taught to children, including "prehomosexual" children, at a very early age. The term *internalized homophobia* is often used to refer to antihomosexual bias that is absorbed from parents and peers and penetrates deep into the developing psyche, sometimes festering for many years, before suddenly inflicting damage during adolescence or adulthood. (More about this in a later chapter.)

Many gay and lesbian adults can often recall having had attractions to same-sex peers as younger children which, though not sexual, seem compelling and intense: "Oh, what I would have given to be Tommy's real best friend. God, how I wanted to be *like* him, to do the same mischievous, self-assured things he did, to have muscles and blond hair and a smile like his . . . just to be like the Hardy Boys, two blood brothers, two cowboys—that's it: two *cowboys.*"[5] Not enough research has been done to determine whether there is a qualitative difference between these relationships and the intense childhood bondings that heterosexual adults also report. Nevertheless, reports of these kinds of admirations may well represent another aspect of the "sensitization" of the "prehomosexual" to same-sex attraction later in life.

In adolescence, the individual first comes to mull over the possibility that some of his or her feelings might be regarded as homosexual. For the first time the feeling of being different from same-sex peers begins to include a feeling of being *sexually* different. At age twelve or so, young people begin to develop an awareness of sexual signals in the world around them.

A former professor of mine tells a story to illustrate this transition, describing an incident in which he took along his two young sons to the auto shop to drop off the family car for some repairs. Tacked to the wall over the service manager's podium was an erotic pinup picture of a young woman. The professor's younger son, a boy of seven or so, noticed the picture but didn't seem to find it particularly interesting. The twelve-year-old boy, on the other hand, found the picture positively arresting, enthusiastically trying to engage his embarrassed dad in a discussion of who this woman was, why she had no clothes on, and why the picture was there in the first place. Although children are surrounded by sexual signals all the time, the message from the signals doesn't become personally relevant, let alone compelling, until puberty.

Adolescents notice the physical changes in their bodies and the bodies of their peers and compare their developmental progress. An intense preoccupation with clothing and grooming is a reflection of a more private preoccupation with breast or musculature development, beard growth, pubic hair development, genitalia growth. Constantly assessing their peers' progress, adolescents compare their own and draw conclusions. They compare their feelings and behaviors as well as physical attributes. Boys notice their peers' expressions of admiration for an attractive girl. Girls discuss which boys are "cute." The discussions soon become more frankly sexual, and the appeal of particular sexual behaviors with particular partners is enthusiastically debated. The bolder ones soon begin to boast of sexual encounters.

Some adolescents begin to recognize an incongruity between their own feelings and those reported by their peers. This incongruity may take the form of a lack of the intense interest in the opposite sex reported by peers, or an awareness of an interest in members of the same sex, or both. By now having accumulated at least some knowledge of the meaning of homosexuality, the adolescent acquires an awareness that this phenomenon may have personal relevance. This second stage of identity development has been called "identity confusion."[6] "You are not sure who you are. You are confused about what sort of person you are and where your life is going. You ask yourself 'Who am I?' 'Am I a homosexual?' 'Am I really a heterosexual?' "[7]

Research done in the 1970s indicated that adolescents enter this stage prior to age fifteen,[8] and more recent work seems to indicate that this age is dropping, perhaps as a result of the increasing amounts of information about homosexuality available now.[9] A number of factors are responsible for the confusion experienced during this time, and they often prevent an easy resolution of these questions for the individual. Many teenagers experience attraction and even erotic arousal toward members of both sexes. This can result in confusion because they may think that homosexual and heterosexual attractions are always mutually exclusive. The adolescent may be puzzled by inaccurate information about homosexuality, such as "all gay men want to wear dresses and be women." Most of the confusion, however, arises from the conflict between their emerging homosexual feelings and their heretofore lifelong assumption that they are heterosexual like "everybody else."

The stigma surrounding homosexuality which the individual internalized at a younger age adds emotional overtones to this dilemma. The adolescent is confronted by the possibility that a previously held self-image as a "normal" person may be incorrect and he or she may in fact be terribly "abnormal," "perverted," "sinful," or any number of other negative characterizations that spring from internalized stigmatization of homosexuality.

When a person is confronted by two contradictory facts both of which appear to be simultaneously true, a psychological state results which has been called "cognitive dissonance." This state of bewilderment and disorientation is often accompanied by profound anxiety and fear, uncomfortable feelings that cause the individual to try to resolve the situation quickly. Faced with these new and unexpected sexual feelings, the individual is forced to analyze his or her previously held self-image in light of new information.

For some adolescents, the resolution occurs as a flash of insight in which years of vague uneasiness about an undefinable differentness from their peers crystallizes into the realization that they are gay or lesbian:

> I was in the dressing room of the high school auditorium getting props ready for the play that we were rehearsing when another boy walked into the room wearing only his briefs. Like a lightning bolt, this thrill went through me that I had never felt before—I couldn't take my eyes off him. He was a swimmer or gymnast or something and I had never seen such a broad-shouldered, muscular good-looking guy—maybe I just never noticed guys in this way before. It was disorienting—I wanted to say, "Wow, look at this!" but I could tell that no one else was noticing what I was noticing. The other guys in the room weren't having this feeling, whatever it was, so I just sort of looked away. As days passed, I started to go out of my way to "run into" John in the hall and that same thrill would come back if I saw him and if he so much as said "Hi" to me. This went on for a couple of weeks; I was just sort of enjoying these feelings and thinking things like "What a neat guy he is, how lucky to be so good-looking," but I wasn't really understanding these new feel-

ings—certainly not the intensity of them, not at all. Then one day, I was on the subway home from school and some guys were joking around and one called another a "fag." I had heard that word ten thousand times before—but this time it penetrated to somewhere different in my brain. "*That's* it," I thought; "*that's* what this is all about—I'm gay." Finally, it all made sense.[10]

For this boy, this was what Isay refers to as the "Aha!" experience that many gay men and lesbians have: "like the pieces of an old puzzle falling into place."[11]

For other adolescents, however, there is a tremendous struggle, perhaps largely unconscious, to avoid labeling themselves as homosexual. One mechanism used to avoid self-labeling as homosexual is what psychologists call "denial." The individual simply refuses to acknowledge that he or she is having these feelings. There is a separation of the thinking and feeling components of their psychological functioning, and the unacceptable feelings are mentally ejected whenever they crop up—the psychological equivalent of the ostrich's attempt at avoiding danger by putting its head in the sand.

At the very beginning of this stage of identity confusion when adolescents are just beginning to be aware of homosexual thoughts and feelings, they may seek to avoid being forced into drawing a conclusion about themselves by avoiding any further exploration of the issue. They may throw themselves into activities and interests they have come to associate with heterosexuality and avoid those they associate with homosexuality. A boy may abruptly quit taking music lessons and go out for the high school baseball team; a girl may drop off the softball team and take up dance. Changes in social behavior may occur. Eliminating exposure to the opposite sex as much as possible also eliminates confronting a relative lack of sexual interest in opposite-sex peers, which might confirm one's homosexuality. Conversely, adolescents may throw themselves into a frenzy of heterosexual dating and sexual activity and, in the case of females, even become pregnant in order to "prove" their heterosexuality to themselves. Escape into alcohol and drug abuse may serve the dual purposes of distracting the individual from unacceptable feelings and providing an excuse for having them in the first place ("These crazy thoughts only come to me when I'm high").

Some seek to be "cured" of these thoughts and feelings and turn to a therapist or counselor in the hope of having them eradicated. An elaborate network of "support groups" and counselors has sprung up in recent years, almost exclusively sponsored by conservative religious groups, which welcome these individuals and promise to accomplish just what they hope for. ("Reparative therapy" is discussed in Chapter 15.)

Even individuals who have had sexual contact with a same-sex peer during adolescence may use a variety of strategies that can allow them to defer self-labeling as homosexual. Feelings and even behavior can be redefined as something other than homosexual. A "special case" scenario may develop in which individuals redefine their feelings and behavior as a unique reaction to one extraordinary person. They persuade themselves that in any other context they would not have homosexual feelings. The "ambisexual strategy" consists of acknowledging that some thoughts and feelings can be labeled homosexual but maintaining, "I could be heterosexual if I wanted to."[12] The individual takes comfort from theories about sexuality which stress "bisexual potential" in everyone. When confronted with rumors that he was homosexual, singer Elton John stated for several years that he was "bisexual" and only more recently candidly described himself as "a gay man" in a television interview. Although this attempt to avoid being labeled as homosexual by others may or may not have reflected a similar internal struggle for John, it certainly illustrates an effective use of redefining facts to avoid an unacceptable conclusion.

These coping mechanisms can be elaborated and nurtured by an individual conflicted over homosexual feelings for a very long time. Sometimes, there may be an indefinite postponement of adopting a homosexual identity. Psychologist Vivian Cass states that these individuals experience "identity foreclosure," a developmental shutdown.[13] The individual may develop in other ways, but his or her sexual orientation identity stops developing. Considerable psychological energy must continue to be expended denying, avoiding, or redefining homosexual thoughts and feelings (and sometimes behavior) to prevent incorporating them into the individual's identity. Instead of experiencing the increasing congruence and consistency about sexual identity which serve as a basis for healthy relationships, he or she is stuck (perhaps Freud would have said "fixated") at a point of irreconcilable conflicts and contradictions that must constantly be juggled and manipulated.

It is important to emphasize that the development of a homosexual identity and the decision to engage in same-sex intimacy are quite independent processes. Individuals may engage in homosexual behaviors for a variety of purposes. Kinsey showed that many people he interviewed had at least some homosexual experience. Homosexual contact during adolescence as an expression of sexual exploring and defining is common. Teenage male prostitutes, found throughout the United States and the world, exhibit what might be called "economic" homosexuality—many, perhaps most, of these young men consider themselves heterosexual. Homosexuality in closed institutions like prisons and boarding schools has been called "situational homosexuality." When same-sex intimacy is the only available outlet for sexual release, many individuals engage in homosexual activity. For these individuals, homosexual behavior is a kind of detour in their development of a heterosexual identity. Often, the homosexual activity is accompanied by fantasies of heterosexual activity.

Teenage heterosexual males may have occasional thoughts about performing oral sex on another male or being anally penetrated by one, but these fantasies seem foreign to them and are often distressing. Other boys, though perhaps distressed because these fantasies are unwanted, find thinking about sex with men arousing and find themselves thinking about male bodies during masturbation. For the majority of individuals, sexual fantasies and feelings increasingly center on males or on females during adolescence, and assigning meaning to them in terms of a sexual orientation identity can occur independently of physical sexual activity.

Many, perhaps even most, homosexuals go through at least a brief period of cognitive dissonance and some psychological gymnastics before they reach a point of acceptance or at least tolerance of the label *homosexual* as applied to themselves. But once this point is reached, yet another crossroads presents itself: will the individual allow others to perceive him or her as homosexual? Now the individual enters a different phase of identity development altogether. Where the first part of the process was characterized mostly by internal psychological processes, the second part is concerned much more with external forces, society and culture. To understand this next part of identity development, a solid understanding of another phenomenon is needed. In the next chapter, we'll learn about stigma and its management.

TWELVE

Stigma Management

In a 1963 essay now considered a classic, sociologist Erving Goffman discussed the phenomenon of bigotry and the process of discrimination. He introduced his thoughts with a grisly explanation of the origin of the word *stigma*: "The Greeks, who were apparently strong on visual aids, originated the term *stigma* to refer to bodily signs designed to expose something unusual and bad about the moral status of the signifier. The signs were cut or burnt into the body and advertised that the bearer was a slave, a criminal, or a traitor—a blemished person, ritually polluted, to be avoided, especially in public places."[1] Persons who are members of a group considered "unusual" or morally "bad" are still referred to as sharing a "stigma" or being "stigmatized." The process of labeling them so and treating them differently than "normals" is called "stigmatization."

Goffman noted that in some cases the bodily sign of a person's particular "stigma" is absent. If the "visual aid" is missing, the stigma is, at first, invisible. Unlike those stigmatized by their skin color or physical impairment, these persons are treated as "polluted" only if their invisible stigma is somehow revealed. Invisible stigmatized conditions include "the blemishes of individual character . . . domineering or unnatural passions, treacherous and rigid beliefs . . . mental disorder, imprisonment, addiction, alcoholism, homosexuality, unemployment and radical political behavior."[2]

In the more than thirty years since this essay was written, many of the conditions on this list have come to be significantly less stigmatized. With the possible exception of "imprisonment," only homosexuality is still considered to be a reason for "normals" to avoid, exclude, and even persecute the individuals so designated. Although homosexuality is much less stigmatized than it was only a few years ago, much stigmatization remains: more than half of the states in this country continue to define private consensual sexual contact between same-sex adult partners as a criminal activity. Certain occupations are completely off-limits for openly gay or lesbian individuals: the military, of course, and law enforcement positions in some communities. Sometimes homosexuals are banned explicitly; other times rules and regulations addressing employees who are threats to morale, discipline, or even an "orderly workplace" are invoked to get rid of those discovered to be homosexual. Many churches condemn homosexuality explicitly (some have more recently adopted the position of condemning homosexual behavior only and distancing themselves from condemnations of individuals). The reasons for and the dynamics of stigmatization will be explored in Chapter 14. Suffice it to say that homosexuality continues to be viewed as undesirable by many in our society and there are negative consequences of being identified as homosexual.

Homosexuality is, however, invisible. The homosexual can escape the consequences of being identified as a member of the stigmatized group by controlling others' access to information about him or her. The ability to control information introduces a whole new set of complexities for the individual: quoting Goffman again, "To tell or not to tell; to let on or not to let on; to lie or not to lie; and in each case, to whom, how, when and where?"[3]

To take up the discussion of homosexual identity development once more, after an individual reaches the point of self-labeling as homosexual (the stage of "identity acceptance" as proposed by Troiden and Cass and described in the last chapter), he or she must decide how to fit this information into other aspects of life. External hazards as well as residual internalized stigmatization of homosexuality conspire to make this a difficult process for some.

Some homosexual individuals face a whole variety of risks from their environment: risks of losing their job, being thrown out of the house by parents, being beaten up by schoolmates, being passed over for a promotion (the so-called lavender ceiling), being shunned by their church congregation. But internalized stigmatization (also called internalized homophobia) can also cause pain: an *expectation* of being rejected by friends, feelings of exclusion from the "heterosexual" world of opposite-sex dating, marriage, parenthood. Feelings of shame and embarrassment at the prospect of being identified as gay or lesbian are the most common manifestations of internalized stigmatization of homosexuality. Being identified as a gay or lesbian in any particular setting means not only facing possible threats from without but also possibly triggering the emergence of painful feelings within. To face these external and internal threats to well-being, the developing individual evolves a repertoire of techniques for stigma management.

It should be emphasized that models of homosexual identity development are like maps of a newly explored continent: incomplete and oversimplified. The tremendous variation among individuals and their families and communities will result in tremendous variation in an individual's developmental experiences. Many individuals quickly and easily become settled in their sexual orientation identity and confidently start communicating this identity to others immediately. For others the process is slower and more difficult. At any point, there is the possibility of "identity foreclosure"—the developmental shutdown that happens if personal growth in sexual orientation development ceases and the individual instead expends psychological energies juggling conflicts and avoiding unpleasant feelings.

Some individuals may decide that the consequences of being identified as homosexual are so terrible that no disclosure is possible. The individual might project an "asexual" identity to the world rather than face the consequences of being identified as homosexual, a coping strategy that has been called "capitulation."[4]

Passing as heterosexual is another strategy for stigma management. These individuals self-define as gay or lesbian but conceal their homosexuality from others. At the most extreme, these individuals lead double lives, actively nurturing the appearance of heterosexuality by misrepresentation and lies if necessary. They must expend tremendous energy keeping their homosexual and heterosexual lives separate, constantly guarding against being seen in the wrong place with the wrong person.

As individuals become more comfortable with their homosexuality, they move into a stage where they do not merely tolerate their homosexual identity but begin to accept this view of themselves as a valid, meaningful, and fulfilling self-identity. Terms like *commitment* and *acceptance* have been applied to this stage. Exposure to other gay and lesbian persons seems to be very important for individuals to reach this stage of development. Only with an awareness of the details of homosexual lives as they are lived by real men and women can individuals come to accept a homosexual identity as valid. Changes in our society over the last decade or so have made this much more possible for individuals at younger and younger ages. Where once the only homosexual "culture" was that of the gay bar, now entire communities of gay and lesbian people with every type of cultural institution can be found in larger cities all over the world. Anthropologist Gilbert Herdt has emphasized the impact that these communities have on the development of homosexual identity for today's young people:

> Gay professional and political action groups [appeared during the 1980s and were] reported upon in a plethora of newly founded gay and lesbian newspapers and related periodicals, some produced by local gay organizations. New gay and lesbian religious groups sprang up. Gay merchants and shops emerged and appealed to gay and lesbian clientele. . . . Gay academic unions, social clubs, networks of artists, and special interest groups appeared as never before, providing unprecedented channels of communication and interaction with others in one's city and elsewhere.[5]

These developments have made it much easier for gay and lesbian adolescents to become aligned with a group of persons they can identify with, soothing the dreadful feelings of isolation which trouble so many of them. The increasing numbers of sympathetically portrayed gay and lesbian characters in films and on television also help. These external factors allow the individual to appreciate a homosexual self-identity as a valid one and foster internal changes. A consolidation of the sexual with the romantic aspects of relationships occurs, redefining the same sex as a legitimate source of love and affection, not only of sexual gratification. Acknowledging "falling in love" with a same-sex individual is a sign of deep commitment to a homosexual identity (after all, homosexuality is more about love than it is about sex). Individuals express higher degrees of happiness and satisfaction and are less troubled by internal conflict.

Soon, the individual grows impatient with stigma management:

There was this guy in the office who was constantly gay-bashing—calling someone a "fag" behind their back, telling jokes about "queers" and "dykes." One time in the lounge another guy said that he thought the jokes were "offensive" and Dan said to him, "What's the problem, Tim, I thought you were married, or do you like to swing both ways?" Well, I had only been working there for two weeks—and I'd never done anything like it before, but before I knew what I was doing, I heard myself saying, "No, Dan, Tim's not gay, but I'm a lesbian and if I hear one more 'dyke' joke from you, I'm reporting you to Human Resources for sexual harassment." There were six people in the lounge, so the number of persons on the planet who knew I was gay had just doubled—but I didn't care. I felt great. All of a sudden I understood why people march in gay pride parades. What a rush![6]

As individuals incorporate their sexual orientation identity into the totality of their image of themselves, they become aware of another incongruity: that between the positive attitudes about homosexuality which they are developing and society's often critical and disparaging attitudes. "Passing," with its dependence on covertness, becomes more and more unacceptable. Increasingly, the individual uses disclosure of homosexuality as a strategy for coping.

Sometimes, a combination of pride and anger leads to defiance and desire for confrontation for some individuals (a stage called "identity pride" by Cass). It is possible for these individuals to develop the unhealthy view of a world divided into the "good" (gay) and the "bad" (nongay). These individuals may totally immerse themselves in a gay and lesbian community in a large city and avoid contact with heterosexuals as much as possible. Heterosexuals (sometimes disparagingly called "breeders") and heterosexual institutions, such as marriage, are devalued and gay institutions idealized. The assumption may be that all heterosexuals are bigots and that the only true source of emotional fulfillment is other gays and lesbians. This is a type of identity foreclosure too. If such an individual has contact with a nongay person who is affirming of the former's homosexual orientation, it throws an element of incongruity into his or her neat division of people into good guys and bad guys based on sexual orientation. Rationalizations and even a little paranoia are required to maintain the status quo. ("Your brother acts like he's supportive to your face, but I bet he calls you 'my brother the fag' in front of his redneck friends!") In cities with large gay communities where total immersion and isolation in a homosexual subculture is possible, foreclosure at the "Pride" stage can last for a long time.

As a person's sexual orientation is integrated into his or her fuller identity, homosexuality becomes a less prominent part of the self-image. With increasing maturity, any rigid isolationist attitudes soften. Any antihomosexual bigotry experienced in society is less personalized and is less threatening because these individuals have developed a richer, more complex self-image of which sexual orientation is only one part. Self-disclosure becomes more automatic—in fact, increasingly unnecessary because the person's homosexuality becomes public knowledge in family, social, and work settings. This fusion of the individual's private and public identity into one makes the manipulations of "passing" unnecessary. Happiness and well-being increase as the psychological energy that had been expended on coping mechanisms becomes free for greater psychological growth.

It would be wise to emphasize again that this developmental process differs enormously from one individual to another and that no model can encompass the almost infinite range of possible human experiences. Special discussion is warranted, for example, concerning the differences in homosexual identity development between men and women. Psychological and sociological research has revealed that sexual orientation identities are more fluid in at least some women than they are in men.[7] Erotic attraction and sexual behavior seem less important and affection and emotional bonding more important in women's relationships as compared with those of men. Numerous studies have shown that women have much more "cross-preference" sexual fantasy than men do.[8] Perhaps because of these factors, as well as other unknown ones, sexual orientation identity appears to develop according to less rigid timetables in women compared with in men and to be more strongly shaped by relationship experiences. In one study, when a large group of individuals were asked to rate themselves on the Kinsey scale, more women than men rated themselves toward the middle of the scale and reported more significant shifts along the continuum during their lifetime.[9]

One psychologist has even proposed that women identifying themselves as lesbians can be subdivided into "primary" and "elective" lesbians.[10] Primary lesbians experience their sexual orientation as beyond their control. They more frequently report feeling different from other girls as children, and they clearly identify this difference as one of sexual attraction and orientation. Elective lesbians perceive their identity as more consciously chosen and do not recall feeling different from their peers as children. Primary lesbians would thus be expected to experience the kind of developmental processes and stages which are discussed in the paragraphs above, whereas the elective lesbians would have much more complex and perhaps varied developmental experiences—experiences for which the developmental model discussed above might be largely irrelevant.[11]

Adolescents identifying themselves as gay must face the frightening realities of the AIDS epidemic. Misconceptions about AIDS—that it is exclusively a "gay disease" or an inevitable consequence of a homosexual identity—can add to these adolescents' developmental conflicts and may lead to identity foreclosure. In an article on homosexual adolescents, one researcher reports with dismay the words of one gay teenager, "I never wanted to be gay. Now, with AIDS, I have even less reason to feel positive about that part of myself."[12] The special vulnerabilities of homosexual adolescents to psychological denial regarding their sexuality may put them at greater risk for disease transmission than their heterosexual peers. Just as adolescents can deny or explain away homosexual feelings during early phases of identity development, they may avoid confronting the reality of the risks of their sexual experimentation. School-based AIDS-prevention programs rarely address homosexuality, and since gay adolescents often do not yet identify with adult gay communities, they may not benefit from the education programs, condom distribution programs, and other prevention initiatives that those communities have mounted. The resulting vacuum of knowledge puts the homosexual adolescent, especially the young gay male, at special risk for acquiring HIV. Fortunately, there is an increased awareness of the needs of gay and lesbian students in the junior high and high school years. This awareness has led at least some school systems to develop special AIDS prevention programs for gay and lesbian adolescents and young adults. A welcome accompaniment of such programs is the attention paid to the special developmental difficulties these adolescents face.[13]

Research has also demonstrated that the process of sexual orientation development differs significantly between members of different ethnic groups and different socioeconomic groups.[14] Despite variations and differences among different groups, it is quite clear that access to accurate information about homosexuality, positive role models, and a nonstigmatizing environment make the sometimes painful process of homosexual identity development less traumatic. Isolation, exposure to exclusively negative stereotypes of homosexuals, and highly stigmatizing families and communities make the process prolonged and difficult and the individual more vulnerable to identity foreclosure.

For many years, the phrase "coming out of the closet" has been applied to the act of revealing one's homosexuality to others. "In the closet" and "closet queen" refer to individuals who are secretive about their homosexual orientation. "Coming out" has now found its way into dictionaries, the media, and everyday conversation. A 1993 article in the *Harvard Business Review* titled "Is This the Right Time to Come Out?" explores the questions a conservative corporation faces when "the star employee is gay and wants to bring his partner to a company/client function."[15] As the foregoing makes clear, however, coming out is not a discrete event but a process. Like many aspects of personal identity development, it is a process one never entirely finishes.

In older textbooks of psychiatry, the term *homosexual panic* is listed in discussions of psychiatric emergencies. This term referred to an acute psychological crisis experienced by individuals when they suddenly confront the possibility that they might be homosexual, perhaps after a same-sex encounter. The concept postulated that the sudden shift in perceptions of self-identity (from "I'm heterosexual" to "I might be homosexual") causes an acute identity crisis, a disintegration of self-image, causing individuals to become acutely suicidal, even psychotic. The term has dropped out of use as research has shown that such self-discovery is most often the result of many steps in a long developmental process over a long period of time. Even when there is a sudden shift in self-concept, it happens to a "sensitized" individual and not in an emotional vacuum. As noted above, this "Aha!" event is often experienced with a sense of relief. A study from South Africa (where homosexuality is even more stigmatized than in the United States) from the early 1990s found that fewer than 50 percent of a group of gay men interviewed experienced a disturbing "crisis" during their coming out process.[16]

What does this research in homosexual identity development tell us about the nature and origins of homosexuality? It's difficult not to notice the similarity of the models that have been described from different researchers. A presexual stage of being aware of a differentness from peers is followed by the emergence of same-sex erotic feelings in early puberty, negotiation of internalized stigmatization, self-labeling, and finally "coming out." Different models use different labels, often depending on whether the author has a background in psychology, sociology, or anthropology, but the process described seems virtually the same.

The unique developmental processes of gay and lesbian individuals must be understood in order to appreciate them as individuals and understand their lives. The concepts of internalized antihomosexual bias, stigma management, and "coming out" are crucial aspects of understanding homosexuality. It is also important to understand what homosexuality is *not*. In the next chapter, we'll explore bisexual and transgender identities.

THIRTEEN

Bisexual and Transgender Identities

On a bright, sunny Sunday morning in the spring of 1993, hundreds of thousands of people marched along Pennsylvania Avenue in an event most of the media called the "1993 Gay Rights March" or the "Gay and Lesbian March on Washington." The official logo of the march, which appeared on buttons and tee shirts, read, "The 1993 March on Washington for Lesbian, Gay and Bi[sexual] Equal Rights and Liberation." Those who read their program notes carefully also noticed that organizers had taken pains to include *transgendered* people in the various programs. What are these other identities?

The concept of bisexuality initially seems easy to grasp: individuals who are sexually attracted to both sexes are bisexual. But, as we shall see, the more closely one looks at this seemingly simple-to-define category, the fuzzier its boundaries become and the foggier its relationship to homosexuality.

Transgender is a term that has come to be used to encompass several different types of sexual identities and sets of behaviors that involve taking on the attributes of the opposite sex: individuals who express a desire to become the opposite sex (transsexuals) and individuals who dress in the clothing of the opposite gender (transvestites). As we shall see, many different types of behaviors are included when this term is used.

In this chapter we shall explore these phenomena and their relationship—or lack thereof—to homosexuality.

Bisexuality

Where does the term *bisexual* fit into a discussion of sexual identities? Is bisexuality a discrete category of sexual functioning? Or is it, rather, as Alfred Kinsey theorized, a point on a continuum? Kinsey emphasized that any form of sexual activity—from masturbation to homosexuality to sexual contact with animals—"originates in the relatively simple mechanisms which provide for erotic response when there are sufficient physical or psychic stimuli." He felt that categorization of individuals according to whom they had sex with was meaningless. In one of the most frequently quoted sections from *Sexual Behavior in the Human Male*, Kinsey stated:

> [Individuals] do not represent two discrete populations, heterosexual and homosexual. The world is not to be divided into sheep and goats. Not all things are all black nor all white. . . . Nature rarely deals with discrete categories. Only the human mind invents categories and tries to force facts into separated pigeon-holes. The living world is a continuum in each and every one of its aspects.[1]

Earlier sexologists had come to a different way of conceptualizing their observations that some men and women are sexually attracted to members of either sex. Krafft-Ebing used the term *psychical hermaphroditism*, and Havelock Ellis advanced the term *bisexual* in his writings. Both had the turn-of-the-century enthusiasm for diagnostic categories of sexual variations. Kinsey, on the other hand, swept aside categories of sexuality, emphasizing instead that all persons had the potential for an infinite variety of sexual expressions. Kinsey and others proposed that an individual's "heterosexual potential" and "homosexual potential" were mixed and blended by the individual's upbringing, family dynamics, community, and early sexual experiences. Just as it's possible to adjust hot and cold water faucets to produce unlimited gradations of water temperature from very hot to very cold, Kinsey thought any mixture of sexual orientation was possible. This line of reasoning led him to develop his seven-point scale for rating individuals on a heterosexual/homosexual continuum. Sigmund Freud, too, proposed that "every human being is bisexual . . . and their libido is distributed . . . over objects of both sexes." Freud expressed the thought, in fact, that it was not the existence of bisexuality which needed explaining but rather its relative rareness compared with heterosexuality and homosexuality.[2]

Research on bisexuality has been hampered by the difficulty in defining what *bisexual* means. Kinsey opted for a numerical definition: determined by counting the number of sexual contacts with members of either gender. This approach does not, however, capture the wide range of styles and attractions that can be called bisexual. Is the adolescent who engages in sex play with same-sex partners before developing exclusively heterosexual orientation bisexual? The person who engages in same-sex contact only during prison confinement? The individual who is heterosexually married for years but leaves his or her spouse after falling in love with a same-sex partner? These people are all bisexuals of a sort, but they don't all seem to be the same sort of bisexuals. Some researchers have expanded the Kinsey scale to attempt to separate these different types of bisexuality. The "Klein Sexual Orientation Grid" rates individuals according to the seven-point Kinsey scale on their sexual attractions, sexual behaviors, sexual fantasies, emotional preferences, social preferences, self-identification, and "hetero/homosexual life-style" in the past and present and in their "ideal" concept of themselves. An individual will have a grid of twenty-one numbers to describe his or her sexuality—and there will be literally millions of different possible combinations of numbers on such a grid.[3] In many recent research papers on AIDS risk for men, researchers have abandoned the labels *homosexual* and *bisexual* altogether and simply describe "men who have sex with men."

Most individuals seem to be capable of sexually responding to individuals of either gender under certain circumstances, as during the exploratory phases of adolescent sexual identity development and during periods when available sexual partners are limited. Others, however, have more lengthy periods of sexual contact with members of both sexes, and both homosexual and heterosexual attraction seem to be enduring aspects of their identity.

Some of these individuals seem to have a transitional type of bisexuality. They start out self-identifying on one end of the continuum (usually heterosexual) and are behaviorally bisexual for a time on their way to the other end (usually homosexual). One group of researchers interviewed a group of men who identified themselves as bisexual about their sexual behaviors and reinterviewed them one year later. Almost half had moved toward the homosexual end of the continuum, and the researchers concluded that "many bisexuals are in a transition to homosexuality."[4] Several of the genetic studies of sexual orientation in men indicate that a large majority of men can be rated at one end of the Kinsey scale or the other in behavior, fantasy, and self-identification. One researcher reported on the difficulty of finding a group of men who showed an enduring pattern of bisexuality:

> This proved difficult to do. Most of the self-identified bisexual men . . . were in their late adolescence . . . or had a single female sexual partner but serial male partners with predominantly homoerotic fantasies or identified themselves as "in transition" from heterosexuality to homosexuality. Also of interest is the fact that many of these subjects who were self-identified as bisexuals were rated by us as Kinsey 5's (homosexual and only incidentally heterosexual) or Kinsey 6's (exclusively homosexual).[5]

The enduring state of being almost equally sexually responsive to men and women seems to be quite rare in males.

Women, on the other hand, seem to be more fluid in their sexual orientations. Studies indicate that when groups of women are studied, there is a less pronounced clustering at the extremes of the Kinsey scale, and more individuals can be assigned positions toward the middle of the scale. Some women seem to shift their sexual orientation identity over time and even move back and forth along the Kinsey continuum during the life span.[6] These observations may to some extent be explained by the different qualities of male and female sexuality. Male sexuality is more focused on genital activity, whereas female sexuality is more complex, usually more focused on the relational aspects of sex such as intimacy and emotional involvement. This more complex and dynamic sexuality can shift depending on factors other than the gender of the partner:

> Right now, I'm a lesbian. . . . Nevertheless, there are distinct questions, that is, I'm not sure that I couldn't under the right circumstances have a serious heterosexual relationship. I mean, if my current relationship ended, I might be open to men again. My fantasies still sometimes involve men. I've never had any very satisfactory sex with men. But now that I've found my sexuality . . . I think, just possibly, I could have good sex with men.[7]

Although in a group of individuals the likelihood of finding a Kinsey 3 (equally attracted to male and female sexual partners) is higher if the group is exclusively female rather than exclusively male, the number is still small in comparison with the number at the outer ends of the scale. This small number has nevertheless been found consistently in many studies. Some individuals do indeed seem to experience a combination of heterosexual and homosexual attractions almost equally. Two Australian researchers used an approach to defining bisexuality which is different from the Kinsey-based models. They suggested a continuum of "gender-linked" sexuality with heterosexuality and homosexuality at one end (highly gender-linked) and bisexuality at the other (non-gender-linked). Interviews and psychological testing seemed to support this conceptualization in that "personality and physical dimensions not related to gender and interaction style were the salient characteristics on which preferred sexual partners were chosen" in this group.[8] For these individuals, sexual attraction was independent of the partner's gender.

The existence of bisexuality—in all of its forms—would seem to indicate that, as Freud and Kinsey both stated, humans have an inborn potential to form erotic attachments with members of *both* sexes. The observed fact that so few do remains unexplained.

The lack of a social identity for the bisexual person comparable to those of heterosexual and homosexual individuals may play a role. In our culture, individuals with stable bisexual orientations may be influenced by social expectations to label themselves either "straight" or "gay" but not "bisexual." Alienated from heterosexual peers and family because of their homosexual feelings and encountering homosexual individuals who label bisexuality a sign of "lack of commitment" to the "gay community," these individuals may find it easier to suppress their bisexual orientation, adopt the label of "homosexuality," and alter their behavior accordingly—becoming exclusively homosexual in their intimate relationships.[9]

A 1994 study that looked at personality differences in homosexual and bisexual men allowed the research subjects to label themselves as homosexual or bisexual. Individuals who labeled themselves "bisexual" were considered bisexual for the study no matter what their Kinsey ratings were. In fact, more than half of the "bisexual" men had a Kinsey score of 5 or 6 (predominantly or exclusively homosexual fantasy and behavior). The personality testing results led the authors to conclude that the bisexual group was in reality composed of two groups of very different individuals. One group (about 40 percent) showed evidence of depression and reported feeling "troubled" or "not well adjusted." This group was said to represent "would-be homosexuals" who for "various social and family reasons" were "psychologically conflicted self-identified bisexuals." The other self-identified bisexuals appeared comfortable with their homosexual attractions but also had a "higher recognition of their ability to be sexually attracted to women."[10]

Whether or not biological factors play a role as well in the development of bisexual identities is an unanswered question—the research remains to be done.

Many individuals who are labeled "bisexual" can be better understood as heterosexual individuals in unusual temporary circumstances, engaging in same-sex eroticism only temporarily—behavior they will abandon when the special circumstances end. Others are individuals sexually experimenting with different partners on their way to stable heterosexuality or homosexuality. There is a small group, however, who indeed have a "non-gender-linked" sexuality. At present, this group is very poorly understood. Much research remains to be done in order to understand bisexuality before its place in the range of possible human sexual orientations becomes clear.

Transsexualism

In 1966, a psychiatric textbook was published which described treatment approaches to individuals who expressed dissatisfaction with their gender identity. *The Transsexual Phenomenon*, by Dr. Harry Benjamin, brought together for the first time the knowledge and experience, gradually accumulated over nearly two decades, of the psychiatrists, psychologists, endocrinologists, and surgeons who had helped individuals leave behind life as a member of one sex and move into a new life as the opposite sex. The Latin root for "across" was combined with "sex" to describe these individuals, who express the desire to cross over the seemingly uncrossable biological divide between male and female and become the opposite sex.

Transsexualism is a rare condition, estimated to occur in 1 in 30,000 biological males and 1 in 100,000 biological females.[11] The defining characteristic is the desire to relinquish the role of the gender defined by one's anatomy and take up the identity of the opposite sex: anatomic males who desire to have the body and identity of a woman, or anatomic females who desire to have the body and identity of a man. Although individuals expressing these desires had been described for many decades, it was not until the 1960s that synthetic sex hormones became available and surgeons became willing to do sexual reassignment surgery, making something close to physical sexual identity change possible. Christine Jorgenson and Renee Richards were two of a number of individuals who became internationally famous after they went public about their sex reassignment surgery. (Richards had the unique experience of being a professional tennis player first as a man and then as a woman.)

Transsexual persons suffer from a profound unhappiness and discomfort about their gender identity called "gender dysphoria" (*dysphoria* is a clinical term used to describe any unpleasant psychological state). They have an intense distaste for their body, especially their genitalia, sometimes to the point of needing to avoid looking at or touching their sex organs. As children, transsexuals engage extensively in cross-gender play behaviors and often will express the desire at a very young age to change their sex. Boys may make naive statements to the effect that their penis will fall off as they grow older and they will grow breasts; girls may insist that their clitoris will grow into a penis. They take the role of the opposite gender in play situations, boys wanting to be the "mommy" and girls "daddy." Boys may insist on sitting down to urinate, and girls refuse to wear dresses and insist on wearing their hair short and being called a masculine-sounding nickname.

During adolescence, an increasing desire to cross-dress (wear the clothing of the opposite gender) emerges. A recent study from the Netherlands found that almost 40 percent of transsexuals engaged in cross-dressing almost daily during adolescence.[12] As they move into adulthood, transsexuals increase the time spent cross-dressing and devote increasing amounts of their energy and financial resources to the quest to become the opposite sex. They are not usually sexually active as adolescents or adults and rarely even masturbate—avoiding any kind of genital sex: the most vivid possible reminder of their endowed rather than their desired sexual biology. As they move into adulthood, transsexuals become more and more relentless in the pursuit of sexual reassignment, seeking out networks of support to discover the details of surgical reassignment and sympathetic physicians to obtain hormonal treatment. Strict guidelines are in place for selection of individuals for surgery, including requirements such as a year of psychotherapy, up to two years of hormonal treatments, and living and being employed in the role of the desired gender before the irreversible step of surgery is taken.[13] In one large American clinic, sixty-five individuals have been referred for surgery in twenty-three years, only about 6.5 percent of those who applied.[14] As this low percentage indicates, gender dysphoria can be a symptom of many conditions other than transsexualism, including severe personality disorders and even major mental illnesses.

Research on the psychological success of reassignment surgery has been hampered by the very small incidence of the condition and by difficulty recruiting and tracking postsurgical transsexuals over time. In one of the largest studies ever conducted, 62 percent of a group of Dutch transsexuals had to be excluded from the study, mostly because they refused to be interviewed. Of those who did agree to participate, few regretted having had the surgery and most expressed satisfaction with their new gender role.[15]

Studies of chromosomes and hormone levels have not demonstrated anything revealing about this condition; male and female transsexuals do not seem to be different from other men and women as far as their sexual biology (although these studies have been hampered by small numbers of subjects). Many theories, some emphasizing biological, others emphasizing psychological causes, have been offered, but the origin of transsexualism is still almost a complete mystery. Part of the problem in studying the phenomenon is that transsexualism is only the most extreme form of gender dysphoria. There are individuals who have a strong desire to take on the appearance and social role of the opposite gender but do not want to have their genitals changed (the term *transgender* was originally suggested to describe these individuals but has come into widespread use to encompass the whole continuum of cross-gender behavior from "drag queens" to true transsexual individuals).

What, if any, relationship is there between transsexualism and homosexuality? A small number of young persons struggling with homosexual feelings seem to go through a stage of gender dysphoria before becoming comfortable with a homosexual identity. ("I'm a boy, so if I find boys sexually attractive, that must mean I'm really a girl.") These individuals frequently have other problems with self-identity and other sources of discomfort about their sexuality (such as a history of sexual abuse as children) which cause more than the usual confusion about sexual orientation identity.

The most important distinction between transsexualism and homosexuality is that one condition derives from feelings about the self and the other from feelings about others. The defining characteristic of transsexualism is a feeling of dissatisfaction with one's own body and gender role (gender dysphoria); the transsexual person dislikes his or her genitals and derives no pleasure from them. Transsexual persons experience an incongruity between inner self and outer body. Homosexual persons are happy in their gender role, enjoy their bodies, and derive pleasure from their genitals. It is feelings for others which define them: whom they fall in love with.

One category of transsexual persons illustrates that gender role and sexual orientation are separate aspects of self and vary independently: the "transhomosexual." These are individuals who undergo a sex change but retain a "heterosexual" orientation—for example, a male-to-female transsexual who is sexually attracted to women. Although the numbers are unknown, there appear to be a substantial number of these individuals, especially among male-to-female transsexuals. (There are enough, at least, to create a controversy at some lesbian music festivals, where it has been suggested that the "no penis policy" excluding men from the festivals be extended to include a "women-born-women only" clause: to exclude transsexual "lesbians.") Female-to-male transsexuals attracted to men were once thought to be extremely rare, but a recent study indicates they might be common after all.[16] This study also indicated that gender dysphoria, feeling trapped in the wrong body, needed to be resolved before these individuals could make sense out of their sexual attractions.

These findings have prompted the coining of terms to describe the attraction to men or to women regardless of the sex of the one attracted: "androphilia," the condition of being sexually attracted to men, and "gynephilia," the condition of being sexually attracted to women. Thus, heterosexual women and homosexual men exhibit androphilia, and heterosexual men and lesbians exhibit gynephilia.

No phenomenon challenges our notions of sexual categories as much as transsexuality, let alone transhomosexuality. These conditions suggest that the psychological experience of being a male or a female and the psychological experience of being sexually attracted to male or to female persons are separate phenomena and are capable of existing in any combination.

Transvestism

A transvestite is a person who dresses in the clothing of the opposite gender. People cross-dress for a variety of reasons, and transvestites can be subdivided into several groups depending on the function that cross-dressing serves in their sexual life.

For the transsexual, of course, transvestism is an expression of her or his compelling desire to become the opposite sex. In a sense, transvestism is the outward expression of a desire that finds its fullest expression in sex reassignment surgery. Some transvestites are individuals who, while they exhibit some degree of gender dysphoria, do not have a desire for genital reassignment. These individuals request hormonal treatments but do not seek reassignment surgery—although they dress and live in the role of the desired sex as much as possible. The terms *gynemimesis* (from the Greek *gyne*, woman, and *mimesis*, imitation) and its counterpart *andromimesis* have been coined to describe these poorly understood subcategories of persons with gender dysphoria. (As mentioned earlier, the simpler term for these individuals, *transgender*, has taken on another meaning.)

Another type of transvestite is the fetishistic transvestite, or *transvestophile*. This is an individual who derives sexual excitement from wearing the clothing of the opposite sex. (A person is said to have a sexual fetish when a particular object rather than a person becomes the focus of sexual excitement.) The majority of persons with fetishistic transvestism are heterosexual men— there are no recorded cases of the condition in women.[17] These men often cannot achieve orgasm unless they are wearing women's clothing, usually underclothing. Many of these men marry women and may be able to manage intercourse by fantasizing about wearing women's clothing during sex, but their preferred sexual release is masturbation during or after episodes of cross-dressing. In fetishistic transvestites, the sexual drive is detached from the interpersonal emotional experiences of normal sexuality and focused narrowly on an unusual stimulus. For them, sexuality has a compulsive quality, more like an addiction than an attraction, the quality of sexual experience which characterizes a *paraphilia*.

There is some evidence that fetishistic transvestism and transsexualism are related in at least some individuals. Transvestophiles sometimes go through periods of gender dysphoria, and some persons who request sex reassignment surgery have a history of transvestophilia which seems to develop gradually into transsexualism. Some sexologists see transvestophilia (and other paraphilias) as an abnormality of sexual desire which derives from traumatic childhood sexual experiences, a psychological condition resulting from an episode of sexual abuse or humiliation. In *Psychopathia Sexualis*, Krafft-Ebing described individuals with various paraphilias in whom an abnormal sexual scenario seems to have been imprinted on the psyche during childhood by means of an episode of physical abuse or humiliation by an adult. The individual's sexuality becomes fixated on this one particular moment, and some detail—a piece of clothing, the smell of leather, the feeling of being nude—becomes endowed with all of the individual's sexual energy (thus the use of the word *fetish*, originally an anthropological term to describe a talisman, or object of mystical power in primitive religions). Perhaps some crucial juxtaposition of physical vulnerability, emotional trauma, and precision timing conspires to cause a paraphilia to develop.[18] Other sexologists believe transvestophilia to be a variant of gender dysphoria and to represent a sexual identity problem.

Perhaps the most common subtype of transvestism is that seen in the individual who dresses in the clothing of the opposite sex because it is, for lack of a better term, fun. These are individuals whose sense of the theatrical and penchant for mimicry beckon them to cross-dress simply because they and their audiences find it entertaining. Cross-dressing gives the opportunity to ridicule gender stereotypes and question sexual categories in a vivid and lively way—a fact that perhaps explains why gay men seem to have perfected the art form, epitomized by the "drag queen" and the professional female impersonator. (Gay men certainly have not cornered the market on "drag," however—witness the antics of Milton Berle almost fifty years ago and the immense popularity of the films *Tootsie* and *Mrs. Doubtfire* more recently.)

Perhaps the most interesting aspect of this phenomenon is the strikingly different reactions "entertaining" cross-dressing produces in our society depending on whether the cross-dressers are heterosexual or homosexual. In the 1994 Mummers' Parade (a longtime family event televised across the country), a group of men dressed up as Roman

Catholic nuns marched down Philadelphia's Broad Street and gar-
nered scarcely any notice in that largely Catholic city—just another
group of slightly inebriated (and presumedly heterosexual) guys in
costumes having a good time in the New Year's Day parade. The
"Sisters of Perpetual Indulgence," a group of similarly costumed self-
identified gay men who march annually in the San Francisco Gay
Pride Parade, are, on the other hand, frequently cited as examples of
gay lack of morals and profane homosexual decadence. The "drag
queen" triggers the visceral uneasiness about blurred gender roles
which homosexuality causes in many people. For them, a gay man in
women's clothing embodies a rejection of the traditional masculine
role in a unique and very threatening way.

Rather than a reflection of a sexual orientation or identity, transvestism is best thought of as a behavior that may occur in persons of
different sexual identities and sexual orientations. While transvestism
may be little more than an imaginative and lively way to have fun and
perhaps earn a living for some, for others it may be a symptom of more
serious conflicts over sexual identity (gender dysphoria) or of a paraphilia (transvestophilia).

Mental Disorders and Homosexuality

After the foregoing discussions of the problems that transsexual persons and individuals with transvestophilia have with their sexual
lives—these individuals can arguably be said to suffer from sexual disorders—a brief discussion seems in order about the meaning of the
word *disorder*. Until 1976, homosexuality, too, was classified by the
American Psychiatric Association as a mental disorder.

Disorders are characterized by subjective discomfort (as epitomized
by the usual term for a disorder: "dis-ease") or, in the case of some
mental disorders, alterations in normal subjective experiences (as in
mood disorders such as manic-depressive disorder, in which normal
mood states are replaced by abnormal ones, like depression and psychotic euphoria).

The transsexual experiences dis-ease with his or her body and appearance. He or she experiences distaste, even loathing, with normal-
appearing anatomy (genitals, breasts, musculature, body hair patterns)
and normally functioning physiology (menstruation, penile erections,

nocturnal emissions). Sexual reassignment surgery provides relief for some from their discomfort, sometimes to such a large degree that the term *curative* seems appropriate for this treatment.

Transvestophiles often experience dis-ease as well. They experience a compulsive craving for their particular outlet—cross-dressing—which can only be compared to an addict's craving for a drug. They experience intrusive sexual fantasies that disrupt normal psychological functioning and relationships and propel them into behaviors they often feel guilty about. Intimate sexual activity with a partner is not as sexually satisfying as their paraphilic behavior is.

In contrast, the type and quality of the subjective sexual experiences of normal homosexuals are the same as for normal heterosexuals. Starting with Evelyn Hooker, a few brave scientists began examining the psychological characteristics and sexual lives of homosexual persons, and very gradually this truth emerged: homosexuals are no more likely to suffer from mental illness, personality disorders, or paraphilias than heterosexuals are.

In 1976, the American Psychiatric Association removed homosexuality from the third edition of the Diagnostic and Statistical Manual of Mental Disorders (DSM III). In two subsequent editions of this work (DSM III-Revised and DSM-IV), the most important reference book of American psychiatry has continued to omit homosexuality from its list of mental disorders. Both the American Psychiatric Association and the American Psychological Association have taken up nondiscrimination policies within their organizations and fostered research into ways to better adapt their practices to better serve gay and lesbian patients. Numerous books and journals have appeared to guide therapists in helping homosexual people live healthy and happy lives as gay men and lesbians.

Attempts to show that homosexual relationships are "inherently" unstable have never done so. The need of some homosexuals to hide their sexual orientation, and the antihomosexual bigotry that causes so many to be conflicted and guilty about their sexual feelings, certainly propel numbers of them into anonymous sexual outlets and "one-night stands." And just like heterosexual individuals, gay men and lesbians can be unhappy in relationships, suffer impotence and frigidity, become "addicted" to promiscuous sexual encounters, or have trouble with commitment to long-term relationships. But these problems have no more to do with their homosexual orientation than the same problems do in heterosexuals.

It has been said that homosexuality is not about sex but about love. As difficult as it may be to come up with a definition of homosexuality which all scientists in all disciplines would agree on, it seems fairly clear that a homosexual person is someone who falls in love with members of his or her own sex. As Karl Ulrichs said, "Where true love is, there nature is also."[19]

PART IV

Sexual Politics

So far in this book, we have examined the "inside" story of homosexuality. We have looked inside the brain, inside chromosomes, inside personalities, inside experiences and emotions. As interesting and edifying as this may be, it leaves out a great deal of the information we need in order to understand homosexuality—what might be called the "outside" story. I touched on this a bit in the chapters on psychological development when I explored the tension felt by the individual struggling with identity development which is caused by our society's stigmatization of homosexuality. "Outside" influences like stigmatization need to be understood thoroughly if we are to understand homosexuality completely. The manner in which a society reacts to homosexuality largely determines what life will be like for homosexuals living in that society.

Much antihomosexual bias can be understood simply as hostility toward individuals who are different. Feeling threatened and uneasy about the unfamiliar seems to be a deeply entrenched human characteristic. Members of ethnic and religious minorities, always and everywhere it seems, draw distrust and hostility from the majority group because they look different or speak or dress or worship differently. Distrust of and hostility toward those who are sexually different come, then, as no surprise.

Antihomosexual bigotry also arises from the threat that homosexuals pose to a sexual power structure that exists in many modern societies. We've discussed this already as well. We've seen that American Indian cultures that assigned men and women egalitarian roles often valued homosexual individuals for their special talents. Militaristic and hierarchical male-dominated societies like the Aztec culture, on the other hand, severely punished homosexual behavior. We live in a culture that continues to emphasize masculine dominance, independence, and control, and feminine submissiveness, nurturance, and emotionality. Gay men and lesbians embody contrasts and contradictions to these roles, which many individuals find uncomfortable and threatening.

There are internal psychological factors that operate in members of the majority group to nurture antihomosexual bias as well. For example, homosexual men, who don't sexually value what men are "supposed" to value—women—inflict what psychologists call a narcissistic injury on their heterosexual peers. Heterosexual men who worry about their sexual attractiveness to women can be bewildered and not a little insulted by a homosexual man's indifference to women as sexual objects. Put a simpler way: it will make me angry if I find out that you don't care about something that is extremely important to me. Lesbians pose a double threat to the heterosexual male ego, not only sexually disinterested and permanently unavailable to them but, perhaps, perceived by some men as being in direct competition with them for female partners. Antihomosexual bias in heterosexual women can be understood similarly.

We could discuss the cultural and psychological reasons underlying antihomosexual bias for many more pages, but then we would no longer be talking about homosexuality. I want instead to explore the dynamics of antihomosexual bigotry in societies as they affect homosexual persons, the ways in which attitudes toward homosexuals have been manipulated and orchestrated and channeled for a whole variety of purposes—the dynamics of sexual politics.

In the next chapter I will discuss several historical episodes in which bias against homosexuals was exploited for political ends. As we shall see, bigotry is a powerful tool with which to forge political influence. During these episodes, untrue information about homosexuality was circulated in order to persecute individuals for financial gain, for personal vendetta, and in pursuit of power. The potency of antihomosexual bias and the ease with which the unscrupulous have harnessed it for their own ends are illustrated by the destruction of the Knights Templar, the trials of Oscar Wilde and Philip von Eulenberg, and the Nazi persecution of homosexuals during the Holocaust.

Most frequently, of course, the dynamics of bigotry operate to oppress and disenfranchise the stigmatized group. Sometimes the techniques and consequences of oppression are overt and brutal. In 1994, Amnesty International USA reported numerous instances of imprisonment, torture, and murder of homosexuals, including the execution by stoning of a thirty-eight-year-old man in Iran who had been convicted of homosexuality (in *Breaking the Silence: Human Rights Violations Based on Sexual Orientation*). Sometimes, however, the techniques of oppression are subtle, even covert. I witnessed such tactics at the 1994 meeting of the American Psychiatric Association (APA) in Philadelphia. Delegates arriving one morning for scientific meetings were greeted by about twenty men and women (and a few children as I recall) walking a small picket line and carrying signs with messages such as "The Right to be Straight" and "APA, not GayPA." The protestors were the followers of an "ex-gay ministry" who had been bused in from another city to make a political statement. The APA was considering a resolution that would have made "reparative therapy," a form of psychotherapy which claims to be able to change homosexuals into heterosexuals, unethical. The "ex-gays" were objecting to a passage that would have denied them "access to treatment." In Chapter 15 we will explore sexual politics as it operates in our own society by taking a look at two movements that discredit and oppress homosexuals while claiming to help them. Though perhaps not the most violent examples of persecution based on sexual orientation, the "ex-gay ministries" and "reparative therapy" movements may be the most dangerous, because they invoke the authority of religion and science to validate their unproven methods and oppress their victims.

Finally, we will see how homosexual persons themselves entered into the political arena, discovered their political identity, and mobilized their political power. No longer willing to be the victims of "outside" forces, they have become active in shaping those forces to their own benefit.

FOURTEEN

From the Inquisition to the Holocaust

The Knights Templar

We begin this chapter by recounting one of the first times in recorded history that laws against homosexuality were systematically applied for political purposes. This episode, the destruction of the Knights Templar, would become a prototype for other persecutions that followed.

Theologians had written about the evils of "sodomy" as early as the fourth century. It was in the writings of these early churchmen that homosexuality was named "the sin of the Cities of the Plain" for the first time. Throughout the Middle Ages, homosexuality was associated with the peoples considered the enemies of Christendom: Jews and Muslims. Anti-Semitic and anti-Muslim propaganda, often spiced with accusations of "sodomy," was used to stir up support for the Crusades. Lurid stories about captured Christian youths being raped and circumcised during the desecration of churches by Saracens, the "blood of circumcision" running into baptismal fonts,[1] were guaranteed to inspire the local baron or duke to sponsor a crusading knight. How ironic, then, that hysterical charges of "sodomy" would eventually bring about the destruction of the most revered and successful of the orders of crusading knights, the Templars.

The Order of the Temple was founded by a group of crusader knights in 1119 for the purpose of protecting pilgrims to the Holy Land from attacks by bandits and marauders. Leaving behind their families and friends, taking the monastic vows of poverty, chastity, and obedience, these men often led isolated lives in the wild mountains and unsettled desert lands that lined the routes to the Holy Land. Far from being thrill-seeking adventurers, the Templars dedicated themselves devoutly to their holy mission, inspiring all of Europe to donate to their cause. The order became a favored beneficiary of deathbed testaments of devout kings and noblemen (as well as less devout ones who felt they might need some last-minute good works to increase the chances of their getting into Paradise). Although their vow of poverty prevented individual Knights from owning anything except a few articles of clothing, the order as an organization accumulated assets that made it fabulously wealthy. By 1300 the order had 870 castles and houses stretching from Palestine to Ireland, and "headquarter" Temples were established in all the European capitals.[2]

In the later Middle Ages, interest in pilgrimages to the Holy Land waned, and although the Templars' role as protectors of pilgrims waned as well, a new role developed. The Templars were increasingly entrusted by European nobility as guardians of important documents and financial assets. The Paris Temple for a time housed the crown jewels of England, and the Templars acted as de facto state bankers for Louis XI of France and the Queen Mother, Blanche of Castile, Edward I and Henry II of England, and Popes Innocent III and Alexander III. As this role expanded and developed, the Templars came to administer one of Europe's first systems of banking and financial services.

Monastic isolation was enforced by the order's insistence on secrecy for all the meetings of the Templars. Political neutrality and financial discretion were assured by this practice, but so was the suspicion of those outside the order who were jealous of the Templars' power and wealth. The secrecy of the order, as well as its wealth and power, provided fertile ground for seeds of doubt to be planted by a king jealous of the monks—Philip IV of France.

Whether Philip IV inherited the striking good looks that earned him the title "Philip the Fair" from his father is uncertain; that he inherited his father's enormous debts is not. Philip III had battled Flanders, England, Gascony, and Aragon, and his son would spend a long part of his reign attempting to restore financial stability to the crown—by increasingly unscrupulous and dastardly means. Like others who would follow him down through the centuries, Philip the Fair had an uncanny ability to exploit his people's dislike for unpopular groups to his advantage. Having taxed his peasants and barons to the point of riots in the streets, Philip turned to the churches and monasteries, taxing and appropriating until Pope Boniface VIII began to object. Undeterred, Philip accused Boniface of heresy, witchcraft, and "sodomy" to discredit the papacy and exert his own authority over church assets. Abetted by his minister Guillaume de Nogaret, Philip tried to intimidate Boniface with these outrageous charges, but without much success.

Finding the church too big a fish to fry, Philip and de Nogaret, a master propagandist, turned to other, more vulnerable groups. In 1291 (and again in 1311), Italian bankers operating in France were accused of the sinful crime of usury (loaning money at high interest rates), had their assets seized, and were expelled from the country. Next, Philip turned on another wealthy and (conveniently) disliked minority, the Jews. Accusing them of usury and another heinous medieval crime, heresy, he seized their money and property and expelled them in 1306.

Within the year, however, the royal coffers were running low again. This time Philip set his sights on another wealthy group "whose international treasury sat in mysterious splendor in the midst of his capital city,"[3] the Knights of the Temple. Perhaps knowing that, given the scrupulous records kept by the order, the charge of usury would never stick, Philip and de Nogaret accused the Knights of something "too horrible to contemplate, terrible to hear of, a detestable crime, an execrable evil, an abominable work, a detestable disgrace."[4]

The Templars, an aloof all-male society that held secret meetings, was an easy target for charges of sodomy. Philip and de Nogaret, weaving a tale of obscene sacrilegious practices and ritual homosexuality, drew up secret orders for the arrest of the Templars in 1307. In the early morning hours of Friday, October 13, 1307, perhaps as many as 2,000 Templars were simultaneously arrested all across France, 138 in the Paris Temple alone. The arrests were swift and efficient; fewer than 25 Knights were thought to have escaped in the entire country, signifying an astonishing feat of planning and coordination in an age prior to telephones and fax machines. Since Pope Innocent IV had sanctioned the use of torture in the inquisition of heretics in 1252, it was not difficult to extract "confessions" from almost all the French Templars in a matter of days.

Pope Clement, however, whose inquisitors had reported to him discrepancies in the Templar confessions, began to have doubts. Rather than confront Philip, Clement tried to delay the destruction of the order by putting up a series of bureaucratic obstacles. Not a man to be crossed, Philip fought back by manipulating the appointment of a new archbishop of Sens—who immediately ordered fifty-four Templars to be taken in carts to a field outside Paris and burned at the stake. Several days later four more Knights were burned, and for good measure the bones of the dead treasurer of the Temple of Paris were exhumed and burned as well. Clement's halfhearted attempt to save the Templars collapsed, and he issued a decree dissolving the order in 1312.

There is little doubt that the accusations against the Templars were false. Some historians have branded Philip the Fair a calculating psychopath; others regard him a hapless patsy of unscrupulous courtiers and ministers such as de Nogaret. Regardless of who the author was, one of the instruments of the downfall of the Order of the Temple was growing popular antipathy toward homosexuality being fostered by the Catholic Church.

Philip may have been the first but certainly was not the last politician to exploit a dread of homosexuality for personal and political purposes. Eight hundred years later, in an uncanny repetition of the Templars episode, the Nazis would accuse German priests and monks of crimes against Paragraph 175, the section of German law criminalizing homosexual acts, in order to silence clergy who were critical of Nazism.

Homosexuals are not the only victims of antihomosexual bias. When hatred of homosexuals is acceptable within a society, *accusations of homosexuality* provide an efficient and effective means of intimidating, silencing, or even eliminating political opponents, regardless of their sexual orientation.

Two Trials

For several hundred years after the fall of the Templars, persons accused of homosexuality were drowned, garroted, beheaded, castrated, hanged, or burned at the stake in England, France, Holland, Italy, Portugal, Spain, and other European countries. European powers killed native peoples in their American and Asian colonies who were accused of "sodomy." During this period, homosexuality figured several more times in the downfall of the mighty. In 1476, Leonardo da Vinci was arrested based on an anonymous accusation of sodomy which was never proven. Marie Antoinette of France was accused of lesbianism in her trial during the French Revolution.

During the Enlightenment, the number of crimes punishable by death was considerably reduced, and the quasi-religious concept of "sodomy" faded. Criminalization of homosexuality persisted, however; "indecent acts" and "crimes against nature" were the new terms and medical and forensic theories of "degeneration" the new justifications for hunting down and punishing homosexuals.

Underground communities of homosexuals had developed by the eighteenth century, and by the nineteenth century they were firmly in place in many cities. An uneasy truce developed in some cities between police and these communities. Some homosexuals, especially the rich and politically connected, could pursue their sexual lives privately and untroubled by the authorities—as long as they were discreet. They were always at the mercy of blackmailers, however, and scandals broke out with regularity. In 1889, British newspaper readers were titillated for months by accounts of the discovery of an all-male brothel on Cleveland Street in London. The story would undoubtedly have been much bigger had the government not actively suppressed investigations against one of the Cleveland Street clients, Queen Victoria's grandson, Prince Albert Victor.[5] The Cleveland Street affair was a small matter, however, compared with the trials on charges of homosexuality of two men of the highest stature in their respective countries, one an artist, the other a politician. Both men would be destroyed by their ordeals. Their trials became prototypes for a new technique of intimidation through sexual politics—the homosexual scandal.

Oscar Wilde (1854–1900)

By the time he was twenty-five years old, Oscar Wilde was one of the best-known men in London. Having dazzled his professors at Oxford with his literary acumen, Wilde came to London and within months was fast friends with Lillie Langtry, an actress of legendary beauty who had burst brilliantly upon the London literary and artistic scene several seasons earlier. James Whistler, Frederick Leighton, and others vied for her attention and for the honor of painting and sculpting her, dedicating their poems to her, and writing roles in their plays for her. Wilde and Langtry were inseparable and devoted to each other—and quite useful to each other, besides.

Lillie Langtry was intelligent, but she was not very well educated. Oscar Wilde, who took her to lectures and concerts and spent hours talking to her about artistic theory and literary criticism, was instrumental in her success in the artistic circles in which she had suddenly found herself. Langtry, in return, represented Wilde's entrée into these same circles—he lost no time making the acquaintance of the great literary figures of the day. His output of art and literary criticism, poetry, drama, and fiction soared, and within a few years Wilde was a dynamic force in Victorian literary and artistic life.

Oscar Wilde was perhaps the original self-made celebrity, constantly drawing attention to himself with strongly worded criticisms of contemporary society, which he wove into his newspaper and magazine articles on art and literature. His delight in beautiful things and beautiful people and his praise for the sensual and decadent in art were not a little shocking to the Victorians. Wilde reveled in startling the staid with deliciously witty epigrams like "I can resist anything, except temptation" and "Life is the mirror and Art the reality."[6] As his fame grew, Wilde allowed himself to hint about his homosexuality in his writings.

In 1892, Wilde fell hopelessly in love with a young aristocrat, Lord Alfred Douglas. Lord Alfred had the misfortune of being the homosexual son of John Douglas, ninth marquess of Queensberry, whose major claim to fame, aside from being the downfall of Oscar Wilde, is that he developed the Queensberry Rules for amateur boxing. Ironically, Queensberry, like Wilde, enjoyed being the center of controversy and playing the role of maverick. He wrote inflammatory letters to the newspapers and precipitated incidents in public to draw attention to his opinions. He once got himself thrown out of a theater by disrupting the performance of a play whose message he disapproved of.

Having left Oxford before completing his studies, Alfred Douglas had tried his hand at poetry without much success and lived on an allowance from his father. Queensberry was disappointed in and embarrassed by his effeminate son, and Douglas did little to hide his contempt for his father. Though photos of Lord Alfred show a languid young man, often looking passive and bored, Douglas had inherited his father's short-tempered prickliness. Once, after receiving a par-

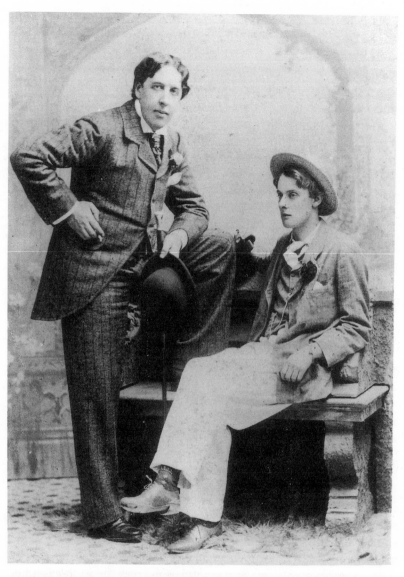

Oscar Wilde (*standing*) and Lord Alfred Douglas, about 1893. (Courtesy of the William Andrews Clark Memorial Library, University of California, Los Angeles)

ticularly blustering letter from his father criticizing his dalliance with Wilde, Douglas fired back a telegram that said simply: "What a funny little man you are."[7]

Perhaps only love can explain why Wilde allowed himself to be drawn into this volatile relationship. In a short time, Queensberry came to blame Wilde for all Douglas's character flaws. Douglas seems to have felt compelled to indulge in anything his father disapproved of—being forbidden from seeing Wilde only caused Douglas to spend more time with him. Queensberry set his sights on Wilde with fanatical intensity, even going so far as to plan a public denunciation of the playwright during the premier performance (attended by the prime minister and the Prince of Wales) of Wilde's play *The Importance of Being Earnest*. Queensberry's plot was foiled when his intentions were discovered and he was barred from entering the theater.

On February 28, 1895, Queensberry left his card with the hall porter at Wilde's club, accusing him of being a "sodomite" (misspelled as "somdomite"). Wilde, egged on by Lord Alfred, made the catastrophic decision to sue Queensberry for libel. Wilde's friends begged him not to pursue the matter, but Douglas threw a temper tantrum whenever Wilde showed signs of relenting in his decision. (Alfred Douglas was not the only one of the Queensberry children eager to take him on. His older brother, Lord Percy Douglas, paid Wilde's legal expenses.) Unbeknownst to both Wilde and Douglas, Queensberry had hired private detectives to scour London for evidence against Wilde. By the time the trial was ready to start, they had found ten young men who admitted to "gross indecencies" with Wilde.

Wilde had the choice of pursuing an increasingly hopeless libel case against the ready and willing Queensberry or leaving the country. Again encouraged by Douglas and, astonishingly, by his attorneys as well, he decided to stand his ground. Halfway through the trial his attorneys finally realized that Wilde would not prevail—that a jury would never convict a father, even the unlikable Queensberry, who claimed to be attempting to rescue his son from the immoral influences of the notorious Oscar Wilde. His attorneys asked Wilde if he wanted them to proceed with their evidence in the courtroom so as to give him time to leave the country. Wilde again declined to flee, accepting Queensberry's plea of "not guilty." The libel trial ended.

By naming ten witnesses to Wilde's homosexuality, Queensberry had provided the state with criminal evidence it could not ignore;

Wilde's arrest for "gross indecencies between men" under the Labouchere Amendment was inevitable. Lord Douglas and Wilde's small circle of homosexual friends, fearing that they might be pulled into the growing scandal, left for the Continent. They again pleaded with Wilde to leave for France, but he would not retreat from his adversaries. An American tour of his new play was canceled. Support among his literary friends, Lillie Langtry included, evaporated.

In his criminal trial, Wilde attempted to deny that he had had sexual contact with the prosecution's witnesses. Perhaps sensing the inadequacy of this tactic, he also pleaded for understanding of homosexuality. For once, he was not merely witty but eloquent. Asked to explain a line in one of his poems, he stated:

> The "love that dare not speak its name" in this century is such a great affection of an elder for a younger man as there was between David and Jonathan, such as Plato made the very basis of his philosophy, and such as you find in the sonnets of Michelangelo and Shakespeare. . . . It is beautiful, it is fine, it is the noblest form of affection. There is nothing unnatural about it. . . . The world mocks at it and sometimes puts one in the pillory for it.

An observer stated that the speech "carried the whole court right away, quite a tremendous burst of applause," and the jury could not reach a verdict in the case. The government pursued Wilde relentlessly, immediately ordering a second trial. Queensberry attended both trials, gloating. He sent insinuating telegrams to his son Percy's wife, a Wilde supporter. Percy Douglas confronted his father in the street one morning and got into a physical altercation with him which resulted in both being arrested.

At the second criminal trial, Wilde was exhausted and broken in spirit and gave no more forceful orations. He was quickly convicted. The judge stated that it had been the worst case he had ever tried. "I shall under the circumstances, be expected to pass the severest sentence that the law allows. In my judgement, it is totally inadequate for such a case as this." Wilde was sentenced to two years of hard labor.

While in prison, Wilde wrote *The Ballad of Reading Gaol*, which was published in England and warmly received by the British press. By the time *Ballad* appeared, however, Wilde, who had been forced to declare bankruptcy while he was in prison, had already left England to begin a life of poverty, isolation, and increasingly severe alcoholism in

France. Lord Alfred returned to his former lover for a few months during this time but deserted him again after a quarrel. Although he had inherited a fortune on the death of Queensberry, Douglas refused to give any financial support to Wilde, stating, "I can't afford to spend anything except on myself." Within three years Wilde was dead of meningoencephalitis, possibly a complication of an injury sustained in prison, at the age of forty-six.

Oscar Wilde was destroyed because he had allowed himself to be drawn into a bitter power struggle between two petty, vindictive men: Alfred Douglas and the marquess of Queensberry. His society's anti-homosexual antipathy fueled his demise, and a law criminalizing homosexuality made Queensberry's revenge possible. Professional jealousy and cowardice made most of his friends and colleagues turn away. Sexual politics had claimed another victim.

Philip von Eulenburg (1847–1921)

Count (later Prince) Philip von Eulenburg was a career diplomat who became one of the closest friends and advisors of Kaiser Wilhelm II of Germany. For much of his professional life, he was the German ambassador to the Austrian empire, perhaps his country's most prestigious diplomatic post. He was mentioned as a candidate for the post of imperial chancellor but declined the position before it was offered. As a nearly sixty-year-old man, he was snatched out of his retirement and put on trial for offenses against Germany's Paragraph 175, offenses that purportedly occurred nearly thirty years previously. The Eulenburg scandal destabilized the Wilhelmine government and nearly destroyed the budding homosexual rights movement in Germany, which was attempting to have Paragraph 175 repealed. At least one historian has theorized that the Eulenburg scandal caused Wilhelm II to shun not only Prince Philip but all of his civilian advisors, coming to be influenced almost exclusively by his military entourage and thus increasingly trodding the path to the Armageddon of the Great War.[8]

Eulenburg was an accomplished musician, composer, and author whose plays were professionally produced in Munich and Berlin. His "Rosenlieder" collection of songs was so popular that five hundred thousand copies were sold in three hundred printings. Eulenburg even designed pavilions for his family's estate at Liebenberg. When the twenty-seven-year-old future kaiser met Eulenburg at a hunting party in 1886, he was immediately captivated by the intelligent, sophisticated older man.

Eulenburg developed an odd set of feelings for the erratic, impulsive Wilhelm, a combination of reverent admiration and paternalism. Wilhelm simply adored Eulenburg, sitting on the arm of his chair like a favorite nephew, turning pages of music at the piano as Eulenburg played. Wilhelm once referred to Eulenburg, one of a very few persons whom the young prince trusted completely, as "my bosom friend, the only one I have."[9]

When Wilhelm became emperor in 1888, Eulenburg advised the kaiser closely on policy matters, appointments, and politics. In 1902, troubled by heart disease and gout and not a little weary of the difficult Wilhelm, Eulenburg retired from the diplomatic corps and from politics, secluding himself with his wife and children at Liebenberg.

Friedrich von Holstein, first counselor of the Political Department of the German Foreign Ministry, was also a powerful man in Germany. Holstein was an eccentric, suspicious man who came to be called "the Monster of the Labyrinth" in the German Foreign Ministry. A master of behind-the-scenes manipulation, Holstein had played a significant role in German foreign policy for years. Constantly gathering information from German embassies around the globe and then sending it where it would suit his purposes, Holstein eventually became one of the most powerful men in the empire. As historian Robert Massey put it, "Without Holstein's approval neither Chancellor nor Foreign Minister would make a move."[10]

In 1906, a candidate for office in the ministry whom Holstein opposed was appointed over his protests, and Holstein threatened to resign his position—a ploy the seemingly indispensable minister had frequently used over the years to bully his superiors. Holstein sent a letter of resignation to the chancellor, undoubtedly expecting that it would never be accepted. But the letter was forwarded to the kaiser with the chancellor's signature, Wilhelm cosigned it several days later, and Holstein was out.

Stunned by this turn of events, Holstein activated his network to discover who had brought about his downfall. He discounted Chancellor von Bülow, who had been home in bed the day the letter had been forwarded to the kaiser. Holstein discovered, however, that Wilhelm had eaten lunch at the palace with his old friend Philip von Eulenburg on the day he had cosigned the resignation letter. Holstein became convinced that von Eulenburg was the man responsible for his ouster and started planning revenge.

Ever the master of intrigue, Holstein had learned years before that Eulenburg's name was on a secret police list of suspected homosexuals and now pondered how best to use this information. He wrote Eulenburg a venomous letter accusing Prince Philip of orchestrating his ouster and making references to Eulenburg's "peculiarities." Eulenburg challenged Holstein to a duel, but Holstein, already working on a more insidious plan, withdrew his remarks.

Holstein had approached one of Germany's most prominent journalists, Maximilian Harden, with his information on Eulenburg. Harden had despised Eulenburg for years, disapproving of his influence on the kaiser. Harden published an article promulgating the idea that Eulenburg and a close circle of friends (the "Liebenberg Circle") "from visible and invisible positions [were spinning] the threads which [were suffocating] the Empire."[11] Later he made even more explosive denunciations, accusing Eulenburg, Count Kuno von Moltke, the kaiser's adjuvant and mayor of Berlin, and three other military aides-de-camp of the kaiser of "secret immorality and unnatural vices."[12] Soon the German newspapers were full of gossip and innuendos against a number of government officials. In a bizarre twist, Adolf Brand, editor of *Der Eigene* (the publication of the fledgling German homosexual rights movement), accused Chancellor von Bülow of homosexuality.

Kaiser Wilhelm was completely outraged and directed Eulenburg to sue Harden for libel and slander. He demanded that Eulenburg return his medals and decorations until the matter was cleared up. A series of sensational trials for libel and perjury ensued from which the crown and von Bülow took great pains to distance themselves. The scandal broadened into a national crisis as more government officials and military officers and families were implicated, including one of the kaiser's sons. The foreign press used the scandal to criticize German society and morals.

Maximilian Harden increasingly became a man obsessed, almost delusional, searching for homosexuals everywhere. He came to believe that there was an international conspiracy of homosexuals, intent on bringing down Western civilization: "A band beyond the divisions of belief, state or class . . . everywhere men of this tribe sit, in courts, in high positions in the army and the navy, in ateliers, in the editorial rooms of large newspapers, in the chairs of merchants, teachers and

even judges. All united against a common enemy. . . . I am determined, with Scythian brutality, to rage against this black band of allied
criminals."[13]

By June 1908, more than two years after Holstein's threatening letter
to Eulenburg, Harden and his attorneys and detectives had assembled
145 witnesses against Eulenburg, who by this time was hospitalized
with chest pains, phlebitis, and nervous exhaustion. Eulenburg's diary
documents the daily arrival at his hospital bed of the investigating
magistrate with new witnesses: "At 5, came the investigating magistrate. Two men were brought to my bedside, with whom, according to
Harden and Co., I had had sexual relations. I had never laid eyes on
them! Thank God, both declared in an oath that they had never seen
me before. What will happen if such men swear they *do* know me? I
am in the power of terrible forces."[14]

By the time the trial started, the number of witnesses had dropped
to twelve. By the end of the first week of proceedings, there were two,
one of them a man with thirty-two previous convictions for everything
from bribery to indecent exposure. In the end, there was only one,
Jacob Ernst, an alcoholic father of eight who twenty-five years previously had been a boatman at the villa Eulenburg had rented while he
was ambassador to Bavaria. Bullied by Harden's attorney and threatened with charges of perjury and imprisonment, Ernst testified that he
had had sexual contact with Eulenburg on a single occasion when he
was seventeen during a boating trip on Lake Starnburg (ironically the
same lake in which the homosexual King Ludwig II of Bavaria had
drowned under mysterious circumstances).

The trial was suspended when Eulenburg fainted in the courtroom
during his wife's testimony. His physician refused to allow him to
return to court, and the trial was moved to Charity Hospital in Munich. Eulenburg required sedation nearly every night and wrote of his
struggle with suicidal feelings repeatedly in his diary. At last, it was
clear that his health and psyche were too fragile to continue, and the
trial was suspended indefinitely. Eulenburg returned to Liebenberg to
live in seclusion until his death in 1921. Court-appointed doctors occasionally burst in on him to examine Eulenburg for fitness to return to
trial, but he was always declared too ill to travel. From the day the
kaiser saw the newspaper clippings accusing Eulenburg of criminal
sexual activities until his death, Wilhelm II never saw or spoke to his
"bosom friend" again.

Historians are divided over whether Eulenburg was indeed homosexual. Correspondence between the members of the Liebenberg Circle can certainly be interpreted as homoerotic, and Eulenburg had intensely close relationships with several of his Liebenberg friends. Philip von Eulenburg's brother Friedrich had resigned from the military after being convicted of homosexual offenses in 1898 (a suggestive fact, given our current knowledge of the genetics of sexual orientation). If he was homosexual, Eulenburg seems to have repressed any homoerotic feelings, perhaps channeling them into his creative activities. He led a quite conventional lifestyle of husband, father, and country gentleman. (By contrast, several of the men also accused were almost certainly homosexual. No less an authority than Magnus Hirschfeld testified at von Moltke's trial that he was homosexual.)

The leaders of the German homosexual rights movement had hoped that the revelation that important government and military officials were homosexuals would help their cause of decriminalizing homosexuality. Adolf Brand's and Magnus Hirschfeld's involvement in the trials backfired spectacularly, however. Harden described homosexual orgies in army barracks and treasonous behavior from effete sycophantic courtiers during the trials, stories that repulsed the German public, damaging the homosexual emancipation movement almost irreparably.

As in the case of Oscar Wilde, Eulenburg had been destroyed by personal and political enemies who used accusations of homosexuality to discredit and humiliate him. As with Wilde, a law criminalizing homosexuality made his persecution possible.

Paragraph 175 was only selectively enforced in Germany, a practice that tempted homosexuals to let their guard down occasionally. When it was politically expedient, a trap could be sprung using information gathered previously. Blackmailing homosexuals was practically an industry in Germany at the turn of the century. (The 1919 film *Anders als die Anderen—Different from the Others*—features the story of a homosexual who is driven to suicide by a blackmailer.)

At the turn of the century, public discussion of homosexuality, like any discussion of sexuality, rarely rose above the level of gossip and scandal—even in Germany, where there were organized efforts to educate the public about sexual issues, especially homosexuality, by groups such as Hirschfeld's Scientific Humanitarian Committee. It has been suggested that as a large middle class emerged in Europe and America during the late nineteenth and early twentieth centuries, a middle-class morality also emerged to define and secure this new group. Strictly defined gender roles and division of labor between the sexes were regarded as moral imperatives symbolized by the idealized family and crystallized in the concept of "respectability":

> Through respectability [the middle class] sought to maintain their status and self-respect against both the lower classes and the aristocracy. They perceived their way of life, based as it was upon frugality, devotion to duty, and restraint of the passions, as superior to that of the "lazy" lower classes and the profligate aristocracy. . . . [Respectability] in interaction with their economic dynamic, their fears and hopes, created a lifestyle that first became largely their own and eventually that of all settled and ordered society.[15]

Oscar Wilde, who had made a career out of shocking the bourgeoisie, of satirizing middle-class values and praising decadence, was the late nineteenth century's sacrificial victim to respectability. Being a homosexual—a sexual outsider—sealed his fate. After Wilde's conviction, London's *National Observer* congratulated Queensberry for bringing down "the High Priest of the Decadents." Eulenburg, who may or may not have been a sexual outsider, served as a lightning rod for growing middle-class antipathy for the decaying European aristocracy. Attacking the kaiser's confidant was an attack on the crown as well, and accusations of sexual corruption among the aristocracy resonated with middle-class aspirations.

There is a legacy from these trials which lives on today, largely because attitudes have not changed nearly enough in the last one hundred years. For many homosexuals their message continues to be to keep a homosexual orientation a secret or stay out of the arena. Sometimes even trying to keep it a secret hasn't been enough. In 1980, eight weeks before the general election, FBI agents walked into the Washington office of Republican congressman Robert Bauman and demanded that he plead *nolo contendere* to misdemeanor charges of soliciting a male prostitute or face felony sex offense charges. An enormous scandal ensued, and Bauman, who had been elected two years previously by a nearly two-to-one majority, lost the election. Several openly homosexual members of Congress have subsequently served and even been reelected. Gerry Studds of Massachusetts, the first openly homosexual congressman, did not publicly reveal his sexual orientation until forced to eleven years after his initial election, again, after the eruption of a scandal.[16]

Although it is now possible to identify oneself as gay or lesbian in many fields of endeavor without catastrophic consequences, in many others, it is not—especially if one's career is a very public one. In recent years, several famous individuals have admitted to homosexuality only after they contracted AIDS. Others, like composer-conductor Leonard Bernstein, had their homosexuality revealed by posthumous biographers. The number of openly homosexual candidates elected to political offices, while growing, remains small.

Individuals who would be famous, influential, *and* openly gay or lesbian are haunted by these trials. Although tremendous progress has been made in opening various public arenas to openly homosexual persons, we do not know how many bright, talented, promising individuals are still frightened into silence or withdrawal by the ghosts of Oscar Wilde and Philip von Eulenburg—and at what loss to society.

The Men with the Pink Triangle

In the late 1920s, a figure emerged who galvanized the German middle class with a vision of a new future. He promised that corrupt and decadent political leaders would be swept away and the wholesomeness of ordinary people would form the basis of a new society. The family, honest work, discipline, and honor would triumph. That figure was Adolf Hitler—and there would be no place in his new society for homosexuals. In the Holocaust, a society's antihomosexual bias would be carried to its horrific conclusion: the systematic identification, capture, and murder of homosexuals.

In 1928, the struggle to repeal Germany's Paragraph 175, the section of the German legal code criminalizing homosexuality, appeared to be gaining momentum. (We'll discuss this movement in more detail in Chapter 16.) Germany's political parties had been requested to give a statement on their position on the matter. The new National Socialist Party (the Nazi Party, for short) made its position quite clear: "Anyone who thinks of homosexual love is our enemy. We reject anything which emasculates our people and makes it a plaything for our enemies. . . . The German people must again learn how to exercise discipline. We therefore reject any form of lewdness, especially homosexuality, because it robs us of our last chance to free our people from the bondage that enslaves it."[17]

A year later, Magnus Hirschfeld had persuaded a parliamentary committee to bring before the Reichstag (the German parliament) a bill striking down Paragraph 175. The Nazi Party newspaper wrote: "Don't think that we Germans will allow these laws to stand for a single day after we come to power. . . . Among the many evils that characterize the Jewish race, one that is especially pernicious has to do with sexual relationships. The Jews are forever trying to propagandize sexual relations between siblings, men and animals, and men and men. We National Socialists will soon unmask and condemn them by law. These efforts are nothing but vulgar, perverted crimes and we will punish them by banishment or hanging."[18]

Delegates from the other German political parties, including the German Communist Party, would all vote to repeal Paragraph 175 in committee vote.[19] Formal adoption by the full Reichstag of a new code that omitted Paragraph 175 was imminent when the American stock market crashed. In the ensuing world financial crisis, the bill was tabled.

In the 1929 election, the Nazi Party gained 107 seats in the Reichstag—destroying any further hope for reform of the laws criminalizing homosexuality. On January 30, 1933, Adolf Hitler became chancellor of Germany. Less than twenty-five days later, homosexual rights organizations were outlawed. On February 27, the Reichstag building was nearly destroyed by a mysterious fire, and two days later a mentally retarded man who had been planted in the building by the Nazis while they started the fire with gasoline and explosives was executed by beheading. During a citywide book burning on May 6, 1933, the Institute for Sexual Science in Berlin was destroyed and with it the largest collection of scholarly materials and case studies related to sexual behavior which had ever been accumulated. Magnus Hirschfeld, in France on a speaking tour, managed to escape with his life.

Hitler's rise to power occurred with the assistance of paramilitary groups who intimidated his political opposition with terrorist acts. One such group, the SA, or Brown Shirts, was led by Hitler's friend Ernst Röhm, the only friend Hitler was known to address by the familiar German pronoun *du*. Röhm was homosexual and not always very discreet, but this fact did not seem to trouble Hitler—as long as

Röhm was a necessary part of Hitler's plan to take over the German government.

After Hitler became chancellor, Röhm's SA demanded a share of Hitler's power—an act that sealed the group's fate. On June 28, 1934, the "Night of the Long Knives," SA members throughout Germany were arrested and accused of plotting against Hitler. Thousands, including Röhm, were executed as "homosexual pigs." Within days, Hitler decreed that the remaining SA commanders were to "take the utmost pains to ensure that offenses under paragraph 175 [were] met by immediate expulsion."

In October 1934, a special team of police was created, the Reich Center to Combat Homosexuality. The same team was later given the authority to combat abortion. In June 1935, Paragraph 175, which had forbidden only anal intercourse between males, was revised to include any "criminally indecent activities between men." The Nazi courts could now call anything from kissing to holding hands to putting one's arm around another man's shoulders "criminally indecent." Any act was considered indecent "if the inborn healthy instincts of the German people demand[ed] it." The Gestapo began to collect existing police lists of persons suspected of homosexuality.

The Nazis had found much of the theory that justified their actions against homosexuals in a 1903 book titled *Sex and Character*, by Otto Weininger—himself a Jew and secret homosexual who committed suicide shortly after publication of the book.[20] In his book Weininger proposed that males were constitutionally superior to females because of qualities inherent in their masculinity. He wrote that men were moral, intelligent, and capable of wisdom and greatness and that women were shallow, immature, and sexually preoccupied—incapable of scientific or artistic accomplishments or participation in politics or government. Men were the natural leaders and women the natural caretakers of home and children. *Sex and Character* predicted that society would flourish as long as these roles were preserved—but would begin to decay if they were not.

Weininger further proposed that each individual's personality was determined by a mixing of "masculine" and "feminine" qualities. While some mixing was tolerable, "intermediate types," individuals with too many qualities of the opposite gender, were dangerous to society because they undermined its "natural" structure. Weininger stated that Jewish men were abnormally "feminine" and therefore dangerous to society. Like women, their sexuality was exaggerated and interfered with the development of "moral sense." Homosexuals, of course, were also abnormal "intermediate types" who corrupted society. While the Jews were not necessarily thought to be more prone to homosexuality themselves, they spread this "vice" within German society to gain cultural dominance. (Nazi ideology also proposed that Jews had invented birth control as a weapon against the Aryan race.)

The Nazis also developed a bogus historical theory to justify persecution of homosexuals. Tracing the origins of the Third Reich back to the ancient Romans, Nazi historians promulgated the idea that the Romans had encouraged homosexuality in the Greeks in order to conquer them. The theory blamed the decline of the Roman Empire on the "spread" of homosexuality.

Using a confused mélange of degeneracy and "racial" theories, Nazi propagandists earmarked various outsider groups for elimination. Homosexuals, Jews, Gypsies, Slavic peoples, criminals, the mentally ill, the retarded, and the physically handicapped were homogenized into a monolithic group that threatened the Aryan race. Words like *inferior, abnormal,* and *degenerate* appeared repeatedly in new policies and laws dealing with these groups. Once they were dehumanized in this manner, their "elimination" became morally acceptable.

The man who directed the Nazi war against homosexuals was Heinrich Himmler. After the murder of Röhm and the dissolution of the SA, Himmler, as head of the SS, became the second most powerful person in Germany. Himmler, obsessed with racial purity, was the perfect person to carry out Hitler's "Final Solution" against the Jews. The architect of the Holocaust, he directed the murder of perhaps eight million people. Himmler's other obsessions were sexuality and reproduction in the Reich.

After the war started, he persuaded Hitler to issue a decree making violations of Paragraph 175 punishable by death. Himmler believed in the existence of an international Jewish and homosexual conspiracy that was bent on the destruction of Germany. Recognizing each other through special powers but remaining unrecognizable to normal men, homosexuals could infiltrate every level of German society and once in positions of power would engineer the appointment or election of other homosexuals. They would then subjugate "normal" men and destroy society.

Lesbians were largely, though not completely, ignored by the Nazis. Like other militaristic cultures, Nazism was obsessed with masculine sexuality and considered female sexuality unimportant. Paragraph 175 did not mention female homosexuality, and Himmler seems never to have made any statements about lesbians. There are a few accounts of lesbians being arrested in the 1940s and sent to concentration camps. By this time, even the pretense of lawful arrest and judicial review did not exist—the SS was arresting anyone it cared to, for any reason at all.[21] One lesbian was imprisoned not for homosexuality but for treason: she had refused to have sex with an army officer.

Since homosexuals could not be recognized by sight, by name, or by lineage, the Nazis depended on informers in order to capture them. Fortunately, the membership lists of the homosexual rights organizations had been quickly destroyed, but police lists of suspected homosexuals were confiscated by the SS early in Himmler's eradication effort. Captured homosexuals were tortured into revealing the names of others—alternately, they might be promised better treatment if they denounced their friends, partners, lovers. Address books, letters, postcards—even a rumor—could result in names and arrests.

Heinz Heger, in an autobiography detailing his ordeals at the hands of the Nazis, recalls being summoned to Gestapo headquarters in Vienna as a twenty-three-year-old university student. Believing that he was going to be questioned about anti-Nazi activities at school, Heinz was astonished when the Gestapo accused him of being "a queer, a homosexual."

> A whole world came tumbling down inside me, the world of friendship and love for Fritz. Our plans for the future, to stay faithful, and to never reveal our friendship, all this seemed betrayed. I was trembling with agitation, not only because of the "doctor's" examination, but also because our friendship was now revealed. The "doctor" took the picture and turned it over. On it read: "To my friend Fritz in eternal love and deepest affection!" I knew as soon as he showed me the photo that it had my vow of love on the other side. I had given it to Fritz for Christmas, 1938. I immediately thought: it must have gotten into the wrong hands.
> "Is that your writing and your signature?"
> I nodded, tears rising to my eyes.
> "That's all then," he said jovially, content. "Sign here."[22]

Heger was immediately arrested and sentenced to six months in jail. Before his sentence was served, however, the laws had changed and he was sent to a concentration camp.

To identify the prisoners in the camps, the Nazis devised a system of uniform markings which used various combinations of colored triangles: green triangles for criminals, red triangles for political prisoners, two superimposed yellow triangles for Jews, one pointing up, one down, to form a yellow Star of David. Homosexuals wore pink triangles on their uniforms.

I will not describe the horrors of the camps. Others have done so much more eloquently than I could hope to. The voice of one man describing one incident will here suffice:

> He was a young and healthy [homosexual] man. The first evening's roll call after he was added to our penal company was his last. When he arrived, he was seized and ridiculed, then beaten and kicked, and finally spat upon. He suffered alone and in silence. Then they put him under a cold shower, it was a frosty winter evening, and he stood outside the barracks all that long bitterly cold night. When the morning came, his breathing had become an audible rattle. Bronchial pneumonia was later given as the cause of death. But before it came to that, he was again beaten and kicked. Then he was tied to a post and placed under an arc lamp until he began to sweat, again put under a cold shower, and so on. He died towards evening.[23]

Homosexuals were among the inmates of the camps subjected to gruesome "medical experiments" by Nazi doctors. In one, which involved homosexuals exclusively, men were castrated and then given injections of testosterone, presumedly to see if their sexual orientation could be changed. The number of men wearing the pink triangle on their prison uniforms who perished in the camps is not known. Nazi records indicate that about fifty thousand men were convicted of offenses under Paragraph 175 between 1931 and 1944.

After the war, the monstrous truth about the Holocaust emerged—but the persecution of homosexuals as part of that truth was largely ignored. The index of the twenty-plus volumes of transcripts and other documents of the Nuremberg Trials does not include an entry for *homosexuals* anywhere in its seven hundred pages.[24] Persons imprisoned by the Nazis for homosexuality were not entitled to the reparation payments other victims received.

During the postwar overhaul, or "de-Nazification," of German law, the strengthened Nazi version of Paragraph 175 remained essentially intact. A 1947 decision of the Hamburg Court of Appeals ruled that the 1935 Nazi law should stand because it had been "justified on objective grounds and thus [could not] be regarded as part of the National Socialist doctrine, so that in principle, no objection exist[ed] to using this new version."[25] Some German homosexuals who had been imprisoned by the Nazis were arrested and again imprisoned by postwar German courts—and some committed suicide after their arrest rather than return to prison, any prison, again. Paragraph 175 was finally abolished in 1969, more than a hundred years after Karl Ulrichs had first begun to call for its repeal, but not before perhaps fifty thousand men were murdered by its authority and countless others imprisoned, before and after the Nazi era.

The torture and murder of so many people because of their sexual orientation—perhaps betrayed, like young Heinz Heger, by a love note on the back of a photograph—is a horror difficult to comprehend. But the deaths of the men with the pink triangles during the Holocaust are unfortunately only one chapter in a long history of persecution of homosexual persons.

Nearly half of U.S. states continue to criminalize homosexuality in statutes not very different from those the Nazis used to imprison tens of thousands of men during the Holocaust. In 1986, the United States Supreme Court affirmed the state of Georgia's right to imprison an individual for up to twenty years for "sodomy."[26] Laws that would make the rounding up and mass imprisonment of homosexuals possible are in full effect in twenty-two states.[27]

The pink triangle was reclaimed as a symbol of homosexuality in the 1970s, appearing on flags and banners in gay rights parades and in the logos for gay organizations, this time signifying the struggle for equality for homosexuals. It has become less popular recently as a symbol for "gay pride" than the more festive looking "rainbow" flag. The pink triangle is too stark a reminder, perhaps, of too horrible a history.

FIFTEEN

Salvation and Repair

Many organizations working today to suppress homosexuality do not advocate violence against homosexuals—perhaps because Americans would not respond favorably to the idea of a Final Solution for homosexuals. More palatable are their seemingly harmless invitations to homosexuals to give up their "lifestyle" and learn to be heterosexual. Two movements have emerged which claim to be able to reorient homosexuals toward heterosexuality, one religio-political, the other medical. As we shall see, their message and their methods are anything but harmless.

Ex-gay Ministries

Six passages in the Bible form the basis for Christian prohibitions against sexual contact between persons of the same gender.[1] Some biblical scholars have concluded that these passages should not be interpreted as forbidding homosexual behavior, arguing that such interpretations rely on mistranslations of Greek and Hebrew words and misconstrued references to Greek and Roman idolatry and cult prostitution for their authority.[2] Nevertheless, many Christian denominations continue to teach that homosexuality is always sinful. Some denominations have started ministries whose stated purpose is to help homosexual individuals conform to these teachings and avoid homosexual activity. Several organizations independent of any particular denomination but with the same mission have also sprouted up. Homosexual individuals who are experiencing conflicts over their homoerotic feelings and who have a need for acceptance by a religious community sometimes turn to these ministries hoping to resolve their conflicts and safeguard their continued acceptance by church communities that would not accept them as homosexuals. Although a few of these ministries espouse the more modest goal of helping homosexual persons remain celibate, many, such as Exodus International and Love in Action, promise to be able to eliminate homoeroticism in individuals and replace it with heterosexuality.

In many ways modeled after self-help groups formed to address problems such as alcoholism and drug addiction (one such organization calls itself "Homosexuals Anonymous," a name derived from that of the familiar alcoholism treatment organization Alcoholics Anonymous), these organizations offer conflicted homosexuals the hope of being "saved" from the sin of homosexuality. A pamphlet published by Exodus International states: "Our primary purpose is to proclaim that freedom from homosexuality is possible through repentance and faith in Jesus Christ as Savior and Lord. . . . Christ offers a healing alternative to those with homosexual tendencies. Exodus upholds redemption for the homosexual person as the process whereby sin's power is broken, and the individual is freed to know and experience true identity as discovered in Christ and His Church."[3]

Like other cult movements, ex-gay ministries use indoctrination and isolation to force individuals to reinterpret their experiences according to the belief system of the charismatic leaders of the group. In lectures, meetings, and support groups, individuals hoping to change their sexual orientation are exposed to tirades on the evils of homosexuality and repeatedly told stories of individuals who have "overcome" a homosexual orientation. Failure of reorientation is blamed on lack of commitment, lack of faith, yielding to temptation, and even demonic possession.

Books, tapes, videos, and newsletters carry the message of redemption to men and women conflicted about their sexuality. Publications by authors associated with these groups often contain "case studies" designed to demonstrate the pathology of the homosexual condition, often describing the lives of homosexual individuals with a complex of psychological difficulties such as alcoholism, drug addiction, family problems, and disturbed sexual relationships. Borrowing from old psychological, especially psychoanalytic, literature, the authors blame these problems on homosexuality.

Stereotypes are quoted as fact. In a paperback titled *What Everyone Should Know about Homosexuality*, written by the executive director of Exodus International and a former counselor affiliated with Love in Action, it is stated that "moral fidelity among homosexuals is almost unknown."[4] "Typical" homosexuals are said to have literally thousands of sexual partners because of an abnormally intense sex drive that cannot be satisfied. Too selfish and self-involved to maintain long-term relationships, homosexuals are depicted as lonely, guilt ridden, secretive, and deceitful. Lurid descriptions of fetishistic practices and pedophilia are often included as behavior "typical" of homosexuals. The threat of AIDS completes the gruesome depiction of the "homosexual lifestyle." These repulsive stereotypes are then contrasted with the serene and unconflicted "life in Christ" that is possible through reorientation.

Aspiring "ex-gays" are encouraged to relinquish their own attempts to control their lives and submit to divine power: "Have you ever given God specific permission to work in *every* area of your life, including your sexuality? . . . Yielding control of these areas to God will open you up for him to work in new ways in your life."[5] And, "God's word—and not my own feelings—determine what is true."[6]

In addition to submitting to "God's will," the homosexual individual is encouraged to practice "heterosexual" behaviors: softball games to help men be more masculine, "make-over sessions" for would-be ex-lesbians to learn how to use cosmetics more skillfully. By acting more typically heterosexual, the "ex-gay" supposedly begins to *feel* more heterosexual: "When I spend some time in the sports page, I feel more informed about what other men are talking about. I feel more confident in being around the 'sports nuts' after church. When I sense their approval and enjoyment of being around me, I feel built up as a man. I feel more masculine."[7] And:

Before I met Sherry, my standard uniform was a T-shirt and jeans, usually purchased from the men's department. Sherry never pressured me to change, but if she needed to shop for clothes, she would invite me along. I'd watch how she combined colors and accessories, and I'd think, "That looks nice." Before long I was trying on clothes and asking her opinion, "What do you think of this?" Now, I can walk into a store and say, "This is me and this is definitely not me." People compliment me on my appearance now; I've developed my own sense of style. Some of my friends actually ask me for advice on how to dress![8]

Word portraits of smiling "ex-gays" with their spouses and children are included as the ultimate proof of the success of these techniques.

The basis of the methods that the ex-gay ministries use to "reorient" homosexuals is an incoherent mélange of theories about the basis of homosexuality—sometimes described in the ex-gay literature as a behavior, sometimes a sin, sometimes a personality trait, and sometimes an expression of satanic forces.

Several ex-gay ministers have been found to be interested in more than the spiritual welfare of their flock. In the early 1980s, a sociologist researching the ex-gay movement interviewed fourteen participants in Quest, an ex-gay ministry that eventually developed into the organization Homosexuals Anonymous. All but two of the men he interviewed reported that they had had sex with the ministry's founder (not surprisingly, none of the men reported any change in sexual orientation).[9] The founder of the ex-gay ministry Liberation in Jesus Christ was ousted in 1974 from the ranks of the clergy of the Christian organization that had sponsored him because of charges of sexual misconduct. The same man went on to found another ex-gay ministry, which folded in 1986 amid allegations he had had sex with counselees. Incredibly, he started yet another ex-gay ministry in 1993 and again was accused of sexual contact with would-be ex-gays.[10]

Although individuals have modified their sexual behavior in deference to religious authority and on the basis of religious beliefs for thousands of years and across a variety of cultures—and few would argue with any individual's right to do so—the ex-gay ministries move beyond an appeal to follow religious teachings and promise to change sexual orientation, an accomplishment that has yet to be proven possible.[11]

One danger of these ministries is that they often blame a person's inability to eliminate his or her homoerotic orientation on lack of will, lack of faith, or, worse yet, intrinsic and unalterable evil and sinfulness. It may be implied or even stated outright that individuals who cannot rid themselves of homoerotic thoughts are themselves to blame for their inability to "change"—and self-blame and hopelessness are a recipe for suicidal behavior. In 1977, a forty-six-year-old man who had spent four years in the ex-gay ministry Love in Action wrote of the difficulties of trying to eliminate his homoerotic feelings: "No matter how much I prayed and tried to avoid the temptation, I continually failed," he wrote. "To continually go before God and ask forgiveness and make promises you know you can't keep is more than I can take. I feel it is making a mockery of God and all he stands for in my life."[12] This man later killed himself with an overdose of tranquilizers and sleeping pills while a patient in a psychiatric hospital. "Counselors" and group leaders in the ex-gay movement often have little or no background or training in psychology or counseling, although they claim to be able to help individuals conflicted in one of the most complex areas of psychological functioning, sexuality.

Some medical and psychological professionals have developed dangerous ideas and irresponsible methods not unlike those of the ex-gay movement. Their psychological techniques for the reorientation of homosexuality are called "reparative therapy."

Reparative Therapy

For many years, psychiatrists, psychologists, and other therapists have advocated different forms of "therapy" for the purpose of changing an individual's sexual orientation from homosexual to heterosexual. Despite Freud's admonition that "to undertake to convert a . . . homosexual into a heterosexual does not offer much more prospect of success than the reverse," entire careers have been built around "reorientation" techniques.

Such claims have made for lucrative personal practices, successful public and professional speaking tours, and scholarly and popular writing careers. Edmund Bergler, a 1950s psychoanalyst, wrote numerous articles in professional journals and several popular books about homosexuality (such as *One Thousand Homosexuals: Conspiracy of Silence, or Curing and Deglamorizing Homosexuals?*). Bergler believed that a pervasive societal unwillingness to discuss the subject was keeping tens of thousands of homosexuals from learning that their "condition" was a "therapeutically changeable subdivision of neurosis" and that "because of an appalling lack of accurate information, [young homosexuals] erroneously consider their homosexual difficulty to be their final destiny" and do not seek out the therapy that could cure them.[13] (Bergler also wrote that the fashion industry was controlled by a homosexual conspiracy and that homosexual couturiers acted out their masochistic fear and hatred of women by designing "unbecoming" fashions for them to wear.)

After Bergler's heyday, mainstream American psychiatry and psychology embarked on a long and arduous process of updating their views on homosexuality and the "treatment" needs of homosexuals, culminating in the removal of homosexuality from the official list of mental disorders of the American Psychiatric Association (APA) in 1976. Unfortunately, therapists who insist that homosexuality is a psychiatric disorder are still practicing, and claims of a "cure" have not gone away.

These ideas are currently embodied in the reparative therapy movement, which in 1992 founded the National Association for Research and Therapy of Homosexuality (NARTH). This organization was started by a group of psychiatric and psychological professionals headed by Charles Socarides, one of the psychiatrists who had attempted to stop homosexuality from being removed from the official list of mental disorders of the APA in 1976. Stating that "obligatory homosexuality is a treatable developmental disorder," NARTH seeks "to counter some disturbing recent developments within the psychiatric and psychological professions,"[14] namely, the increasingly broad-based rejection of the founders' premise that homosexuality is a mental illness. In addition to Socarides—a psychoanalyst who has spent his entire life attempting without success to persuade American psychiatry and psychology that homosexuality is pathological and treatable—one of NARTH's chief spokesmen is Joseph Nicolosi, Ph.D., the founder of a clinic in Encino, California, to which he has given the splendidly appropriate name "Thomas Aquinas Psychological Clinic." Nicolosi has become chief theoretician for NARTH and has published two books, *Reparative Therapy of Male Homosexuality* and *Healing Homosexuality: Case Studies of Reparative Therapy.*[15] Like books written in the 1950s and 1960s by Charles Socarides and Edmund Bergler, these books are collections of case studies of men who came to the author to be cured of homosexual thoughts and behaviors. Based on his observations of these disturbed men, Nicolosi proposes that male homosexuals "suffer from a syndrome of male gender-identity deficit. It is this internal sense of incompleteness of one's own maleness that is the essential foundation for homoerotic attraction. The causal rule of reparative therapy is 'gender identity determines sexual orientation.' We eroticize what we are not identified with. The focus of treatment therefore is the full development of the client's masculine gender identity."[16]

The reparative therapy literature concerns itself almost exclusively with male homosexuality. This lack of interest in female homosexuality among the proponents of reparative therapy is striking but also typical of the reports of reorientation techniques of the past fifty years. All the works of Bergler, Irving Bieber, and Socarides ignore lesbianism almost completely. There are a number of reasons for this disinterest, reasons that have a more political than medical basis. Conservative views of rigidly defined, traditional gender roles drive the reparative therapy (and the ex-gay) movement, views that hold that female sexuality is not as important as that of male sexuality. Since masculinity is the more valued commodity in conservative, hierarchical societies, preoccupation with male sexuality in this movement and indifference toward female sexuality should come as no surprise. Loosely based on psychoanalytic concepts, reparative therapy also shares earlier Freudian theory's "phallo-centric" view of human sexuality (illustrated by one of Freud's terms for the female Oedipus complex— "penis envy"). A more fundamental reason for a lack of writing about reorienting lesbians may be that not nearly as many lesbians seem to seek out reparative therapists. Because male homosexuality has for a variety of reasons been more stigmatized historically than female homosexuality, men may be more likely to seek sexual reorientation than women.

Reparative therapy theory proposes that male homosexuality stems from difficulties in the father-son relationship: if a boy's father does not provide him with an "authentic masculine identity," the boy's masculine identity will be damaged. The damage will cause him to feel inferior to "normal" men, to idealize them and eroticize them. (The corresponding notion, that "damaged femininity" makes heterosexual men feel inferior to and eroticize females, would of course be dismissed as absurd.) The male homosexual is sexually attracted to men because he is (unconsciously, of course) searching to heal his damaged masculinity.

Reparative therapy offers to help homosexuals to heal their damaged masculinity by helping them become more like other men: "Reparative therapy is initiatory in nature. The client must struggle to break down old patterns of avoidance and defensive detachment from males in order to form close, intimate, non-sexual male friendships."[17] Like the ex-gay ministries' encouragement to play more softball, the idea—this time, dressed up in psychoanalytic terminology—is that the patient will become more heterosexual if he acts more like "one of the (heterosexual) guys."

Another theme in these writings is that homosexuals have adopted a gay identity because it "serves as a defense against the anxieties of man-woman intimacies and other adult challenges." In other words, it's easier to be homosexual than to be heterosexual: "Many studies show pre-homosexual boys to be interested in theater and acting. Many of my clients also played piano from the time of early boyhood. I see this as one more retreat from life challenges into the safety of the false self."[18] The author does not explain what heterosexual pianists might be retreating from.

The supporting evidence for these lame theories consists of the usual collection of case studies of disturbed individuals who desire to blame their varied disturbances on a homosexual orientation. Some are men desperately seeking to escape society's and their own internalized hatred of homosexuals by "changing" their sexual orientation. Most of the men discussed in Nicolosi's case study volume appear to suffer from severe psychological problems, such as one who is a recovering alcoholic with a personality disorder, and another who is a man with a paraphilic fetish and bulimia. One of the few who do not seem overtly disturbed is a sixteen-year-old boy brought by his desperate mother to the Aquinas clinic after she has discovered gay magazines in his bedroom.

Like previous psychotherapeutic techniques that claimed to be able to reorient homosexuals, reparative therapy's theory has been derived from the study and treatment of individuals who request a psychological treatment to change their sexual orientation. These individuals have extremely negative attitudes about homosexuality—and about themselves. Rather than help these patients try to discover the sources of their bad feelings about themselves, this "therapy" indoctrinates them with the idea that their feelings of unhappiness are solely and directly a result of their homosexuality. As with other theories that have over the years reported successful techniques for the reorientation of homosexuals, reparative therapy "success" is poorly defined, and meaningful follow-up of cases is nonexistent. There are no controlled studies and no objective interviewers, only the stories of distressed and unhappy individuals desperate to change their sexual behaviors.

Holy Alliance

It will not be surprising to learn that the ex-gay movement and reparative therapists have increasingly joined forces to advance their agendas, which, of course, are essentially identical: eliminating same-sex eroticism from society. The ex-gay movement, while deriving its authority from religious dogma, seeks to bolster its credibility by using the flawed data and unscientific research techniques of the reparative therapists. NARTH, increasingly seeking to portray itself as an organization standing up for "patient rights," often depends on "ex-gays" to take their message of successful reorientation to the public—most vividly illustrated in the incident at the American Psychiatric Association meeting I mentioned earlier.

At that meeting, a "Position Statement on Psychiatric Treatment Designed to Change Sexual Orientation," which had already been approved by the APA's board of trustees, was to have been presented for approval by the Assembly of Delegates. The resolution stated, in part, "The American Psychiatric Association does not endorse any psychiatric treatment which is based on a psychiatrist's assumption that homosexuality is a mental disorder or a psychiatrist's intent to change a person's sexual orientation."[19] This statement would have amounted to an official condemnation of reparative therapy as an unethical practice. NARTH enlisted the help of the Christian Right organization "Focus on the Family" to fund a mailing to APA members protesting this "violation of first amendment rights."[20] "Transformation Ministries" was contacted to supply protestors with placards exhibiting slogans such as "APA, not GayPA." (The position statement was ultimately tabled because of a perceived vagueness in its wording and was not voted upon in the 1994 assembly, an outcome heralded as a "victory" in the newsletters of both NARTH and Exodus International.)

Both the ex-gay ministries and NARTH take as their starting point the position that homosexuality is wrong and that homosexuals need to become heterosexual in thought and action. The ministries derive this view from religious dogma and from biblical passages that are interpreted to forbid homosexuality. NARTH's mission statement says that "homosexuality distorts the natural bond of friendship that would normally unite persons of the same sex. It works against society's essential male/female design and family unit," a justification for changing sexual orientation which derives from the philosophy of NARTH's patron saint, Thomas Aquinas, but could have been lifted word for word from National Socialist (Nazi) propaganda.

Both movements portray homosexuality as negatively as possible. Ex-gay ministries alternate between trivializing sexual orientation with phrases such as "gay lifestyle" and raising Heinrich Himmler's bugaboo of a homosexual conspiracy with references to "the gay agenda." Both movements reinforce false negative stereotypes of homosexuals by linking homosexuality to pedophilia and other paraphilias and prey on public fear of AIDS to justify their efforts. The claim by NARTH that reparative therapists are safeguarding "patients' rights" is especially disturbing. Safeguarding a person's right to receive an unproven and potentially harmful treatment for a "condition" that is not inherently pathological is an ethically dubious calling for psychological professionals to be following.

Statements by confrontational, charismatic reparative therapists that homosexuality is never acceptable and the orchestration of peer pressure by ex-gay ministries to reinforce these statements have the same effects on homosexual persons as the "electric shock" techniques that were tried in the 1950s and 1960s. Subjects undergoing "treatment" by this technique, euphemistically called "aversive conditioning," sat in a chair and watched pictures of nude men and women being flashed on a screen in front of them—when a picture of an attractive person of the same sex appeared, they were given an electric shock. The theory was that a same-sex partner would come to be associated with a painful stimulus and lose his or her attraction. This vicious technique was soon abandoned because it had little or no effect on sexual behaviors, let alone sexual orientation.[21] Reparative therapists use techniques that deliver a painful *psychological* rather than *physical* stimulus—by nurturing their subject's internalized antihomosexual bias. By repeatedly reminding would-be ex-gays that homosexuality is "sick," "sinful," and "abnormal," reparative therapists facilitate self-hatred. Some of these individuals do indeed learn to suppress homosexual thoughts and behaviors for varying periods of time. Those who continue to have homosexual thoughts, fantasies, or behavior despite their best efforts at salvation and repair begin to think of themselves as too damaged or sinful to live up to their program's or therapist's expectations. Anxiety, depression, and even suicidal behavior can result.

In 1992, the medical director of the American Psychiatric Association wrote: "There is no published scientific evidence to support the efficacy of reparative therapy to change one's sexual orientation. . . . Clinical experience suggests that any person who seeks conversion therapy may be doing so because of social bias that has resulted in internalized homophobia. . . . Gay men and lesbians who have accepted their sexual orientation are better adjusted than those who have not."[22] The executive director for professional practice of the American Psychological Association put it more bluntly, stating that "efforts to 'repair' homosexuals are nothing more than social prejudice garbed in psychological accouterments."[23] The American Academy of Pediatrics has also denounced reparative therapy as "contraindicated, since it can provoke guilt and anxiety while having little or no potential for achieving changes in orientation."[24]

By publicizing techniques for the "reorientation" of homosexuality, these organizations have given antihomosexual political groups a unique tactic for oppressing homosexuals. No other minority group is the target of organizations calling on them to "convert" to majority status. The very idea of a movement advocating name changes or cosmetic surgery to help ethnic minorities "blend in" is absurd.

One of the arguments used today by those who oppose extending equal rights and benefits to homosexuals as a minority group is that homosexuals don't really constitute a minority. Their argument is that homosexuals are individuals who indulge in certain sexual behaviors, not individuals with a sexual identity or orientation that is different from the majority. If homosexuality were simply a behavior—especially if it were a behavior that could be changed with therapy—rather than an inherent and unchanging characteristic, minority status for homosexuals would not make very much sense. Although all the available data from the behavioral sciences contradict this view, "experts" from the ex-gay and reparative therapy movements nevertheless regularly appear in the media using their unproven theories and "success" stories to torpedo attempts of gay and lesbian people to pass antidiscrimination laws. Although NARTH communications repeatedly declare that the organization is "for the civil . . . rights of homosexuals,"[25] its officers have appeared in court to testify against legislation protecting individuals from discrimination based on sexual orientation. Reparative therapists and "ex-gays" testified in favor of Amendment 2 in 1994 at hearings by the Colorado Supreme Court. This amendment would have amended Colorado's state constitution to prevent sexual orientation from ever being added to the list of minority groups protected from discrimination. (The Colorado court threw out the amendment as unconstitutional, a decision which was upheld by the United States Supreme Court in 1996.

The ex-gay and reparative therapy movements derive their strength from fear and hatred of homosexuals and do great harm to the individuals they purport to help—as any therapist who has tried to "repair" the victims of reparative therapy can verify.[26] They are part and parcel of sexual politics in the late twentieth century, providing the theoretical underpinnings of the antihomosexual efforts of more overtly political organizations such as the Christian Coalition and Focus on the Family.

Practitioners in these movements increasingly find themselves marginalized within the mental health professions and religious organizations. NARTH members have been kept busy in the past several years writing letters to the editors of professional publications decrying developments like the 1995 decision by the American Medical Association to eliminate references to "sex-preference reversal" as a "treatment" for homosexuals in its policies.[27] Ex-gay ministries are losing members to ministries like the Roman Catholic organization Dignity and Lutherans Concerned, which are working for the inclusion of gay and lesbian individuals in their church communities.

Reparative therapists and ex-gay ministers are in many ways struggling against the tide, which turned on a hot night in New York in 1969 when a riot started in front of a bar in Greenwich Village, a gay bar called the Stonewall Inn.

SIXTEEN

Community and Power

I am an insurgent. I rebel against the existing situation, because I hold it to be a condition of injustice. I fight for freedom from persecution and insults. I call for the recognition of [homosexual] love. I call for it from public opinion and from the state. Just as inborn [heterosexual] love is recognized as just by public opinion and the state, so too I demand from both the recognition that inborn [homosexual] love is just.—Karl Heinrich Ulrichs, *Vindica*, 1865

This clarion call from Karl Ulrichs marked a point of no return in the lives of many homosexuals. Defining homosexuality as normal for them—and not as sin, sickness, or crime—homosexual women and men increasingly rejected their society's condemnation of their sexuality and began to seek each other out. A few who were independent minded and independently wealthy (like Victorian author Edward Carpenter) could live openly in partnership with a same-sex mate—as long as they didn't mind rejection by all but their homosexual friends. Some would even be able to publish their views or their stories about homosexual love, as Virginia Woolf and Radclyffe Hall did in their novels. Less public partnerships existed as well. Mid-nineteenth-century American newspapers not infrequently carried the stories of "passing women," who dressed in male clothing in order to work as men and support their female partners. The truth was usually discovered by physicians attending them during a medical emergency.[1]

For at least a hundred years, the only homosexual "institutions" were those that brought homosexual individuals together for sexual purposes. Homosexuals met in secret clubs, bars, brothels, certain areas of public parks, perhaps primarily for the purpose of sexual release. Increasingly, however, they began seeking a community of others like them, and during the steadily increasing urbanization of Europe and the United States in the eighteenth and nineteenth centuries, population centers grew large enough to support a homosexual subculture in many large cities. As early as the 1700s, London had homosexual pubs ("molly houses"), and by 1914 Berlin had more than forty homosexual bars. In turn-of-the-century St. Louis, an annual "drag" ball attracted hundreds.

Prelude

The early twentieth century saw the first significant attempts at political organization among homosexuals. Karl Ulrichs' lonely but vigorous crusade had laid the foundation for others in Germany, and in 1897 Dr. Magnus Hirschfeld stepped forward to take up Ulrichs' work. Hirschfeld edited the first scientific periodical on homosexuality, the *Yearbook for Sexual Intermediates*, which published the research on homosexuality that Hirschfeld, whose personal motto was *Per scientiam ad justatiam*—"Justice through knowledge," believed would inevitably lead to changes in the law. The *Yearbook* published the results of a sex survey in 1903 which estimated that 2.2 percent of the German population was homosexual—a prevalence estimate very similar to those derived from modern surveys. In 1897, Hirschfeld, a physician, founded the Scientific Humanitarian Committee to advance the cause of emancipation of homosexuals in Germany. The first action of the group was to prepare a petition to amend Paragraph 175 of the German criminal code to decriminalize homosexuality except when coercion, "public indecency," or pedophilia was involved. Within several months, nine hundred signatures were presented to the Reichstag.

The committee was having considerable success lobbying members of the Reichstag when the Eulenburg scandal broke (see Chapter 14). Fearful upper-class and aristocratic homosexuals withdrew their financial support from the organization, and the reform efforts of the committee slowed to a snail's pace. When the Great War broke out, efforts stopped altogether.

After the First World War, other organizations sprang up. Dissatisfied with the scientific focus of Hirschfeld's committee, Hans Kahnert founded the German Friendship Association in the 1920s to provide fellowship and community to German homosexuals. The association opened a community center in Berlin, held weekly fellowship meetings, sponsored dances, and published a weekly newspaper called *Die Freundschaft* ("Friendship"). In January 1921, the association issued a stirring call to action, urging German homosexuals to become more actively involved in the struggle for legal reform: "Homosexuals, you know what the reasons and motives of your opponents are. You also know that your leaders and advocates have toiled untiringly for decades to banish prejudice, to disseminate truth, to win the rights due you—and these efforts have not been entirely unsuccessful. But in the final analysis, you yourselves must win your rights. Justice for you will ultimately be the fruit of your efforts alone. The liberation of homosexuals can only be the work of homosexuals themselves."[2]

The greater freedom of the press that existed during the Weimar Republic led to an explosion of printed material on homosexuality. Thirty different homosexual journals, magazines, and newspapers would be published between the world wars. Books of fiction and nonfiction appeared, as did other works in other media. In 1919, *Anders als die Anderen* ("Different from the Others"), a film starring Conrad Veidt, was made, featuring the sympathetic story of a homosexual blackmail victim who turns to a famous physician (played by none other than Magnus Hirschfeld) for help. A homosexual theater group, Theater des Eros, was founded in 1921.

Storm clouds were gathering, however. In 1920, Magnus Hirschfeld was attacked by anti-Semites in Munich, an assault gleefully reported in the Nazi press. In 1923, a young man shot at Hirschfeld during a lecture in Vienna, wounding several people in the audience. Ten years later, Adolf Hitler would become chancellor of Germany, the Holocaust would begin, and the homosexual emancipation movement in Germany would be annihilated.

The Homophile Movement

The mid-twentieth-century events that destroyed the German homo-sexual emancipation movement laid the groundwork for its rebirth in America. War mobilization efforts had separated tens of thousands of young men and women from their families and communities. Many found themselves transported to the big cities for the first time, often in sex-segregated environments. Those who had been struggling with homosexual feelings alone and isolated in rural areas suddenly dis-covered that they weren't alone after all. As one man recalled, "When I first got into the navy—in the recreation hall for instance—there'd be eye contact, and pretty soon you'd get to know one or two people and kept branching out. All of a sudden you had a vast network of [gay] friends."[3]

For homosexual women especially, mobilization afforded an oppor-tunity to explore sexual orientation identity which would have been nearly impossible in civilian life. Just as Stephen Gordon, Radclyffe Hall's lesbian protagonist in *The Well of Loneliness*, had joined the British Ambulance Corps during the First World War, thousands of lesbians joined the Women's Army Corps during the Second, making it what one historian has called "the quintessential lesbian institu-tion."[4] Relaxing its usual harshness toward homosexuality during the pressures of wartime, the army instructed its officers to avoid "witch-hunting or speculating" and to approach lesbianism in the corps with an "attitude of fairness and tolerance."[5] Lesbians who did not join the military had opportunities to find a community of others as well. The need for women to replace men in the factories made it possible and socially acceptable for a single woman to sidestep dating and marrying, even move away from home without parental disapproval.

At the end of the war, many men and women returned to their home communities—but many gays and lesbians stayed on in the ports and large cities where they had established circles of homosexual friends. A few small, mostly local, homosexual organizations such as the Veterans Benevolent Association, a social club for gay former servicemen in New York, were founded and provided fellowship for those in a few of the biggest cities. There were several attempts at publications such as the lesbian newspaper *Vice Versa* published by pseudonymous Lisa Ben, but most were circulated only among small circles of acquaintances.

The most important "institution" of the developing homosexual community was the gay bar. Although lovers, partners, and circles of friends provided a private kind of fellowship, any real sense of community identity required more public institutions. The bars provided an all-gay environment where homosexuals could shed their heterosexual camouflage and socialize freely with their own. By the 1950s, it was possible for a new arrival to most mid-sized American cities to quickly discover the local gay bar and gain instant access to the local homosexual community.

Visible institutions were, however, vulnerable. Laws against homosexual behavior were frequently and conspicuously enforced in the form of police raids on gay bars, and many of the bars existed only because they were owned by mobsters who paid off police and other officials. Newspaper accounts of police raids on gay bars had the effect of publicizing the existence of a homosexual subculture to the general population—including, of course, other homosexuals. Ironically, police efforts at suppressing the development of a gay community probably had a stimulating effect instead. One effort by police at suppressing homosexuality stirred into action a group of individuals who would found the first significant homosexual emancipation organization in the United States, the Mattachine Society.

In 1952, a man named Dale Jennings was arrested for "lewd and dissolute" behavior after an undercover police officer had bullied him into inviting the officer home. Several years previously, Jennings and several other men under the leadership of Harry Hay had founded a secret society to work for the rights of homosexuals, the Mattachine Society. The group took its name from Renaissance court entertainers called Mattachines, who the society's founders fancied were homosexual. The Mattachines, like Karl Ulrichs before them, rejected their society's view of themselves as defective or depraved and instead defined themselves as a minority group that was being oppressed by the majority. Donald Webster Cory's 1951 book *The Homosexual in America* clearly articulated this view: "We who are homosexual are a minority, not only numerically, but also as a result of a caste-like status in society. . . . Our minority status is similar, in a variety of respects, to that of national, religious and other ethnic groups: in the denial of civil liberties; in the legal, extra-legal and quasi-legal discrimination; in the assignment of an inferior social position; in the exclusion from the mainstream of life and culture."[6]

The Mattachines set out to educate other homosexuals about their minority status and affirm the homosexual identity as a valid one. Recognizing that a life predicated on "self-deceit, hypocrisy and charlatanism" led inevitably to a "disturbed, inadequate and undesirable" self-image, the Mattachines were among the first to articulate the psychological oppression they felt because of a need to hide their sexual orientation. Greater public acceptance of homosexuality would allow the development of a "highly ethical homosexual culture" that would help gays and lesbians "lead well-adjusted, wholesome and socially productive lives." The Mattachines were among the first to speak of gay pride—"pride in belonging, pride in participating in the cultural growth and social achievements of . . . the homosexual minority."[7] At an early convention of the society, one of the founders predicted, "The time will come when we will march arm in arm ten abreast down Hollywood Boulevard proclaiming our pride in our homosexuality."[8]

It was with the help of the Mattachine Society that Jennings retained an attorney willing to make the extraordinary legal argument that Jennings was indeed homosexual but that he had not had sexual contact with the officer and that being homosexual was not a crime. At the trial, the jury deadlocked and the charges were dropped. With this stunning success the organization was propelled into the limelight; membership doubled every month. The society "really took off": "We moved into a broad sunlit upland filled with whole legions of eager gays. Mattachine was suddenly IN!"[9]

Used extensively in publications of the Mattachine Society and other early gay rights organizations, *homophile* was coined as an alternative to *homosexual* to emphasize homoerotic attraction and love (the Latin *philos* means "loving") rather than sex. The homophile movement broadened as more organizations sprang up and newsletters and magazines were started. In 1953, Phyllis Lyon and Dale Martin and three other lesbian couples from San Francisco founded the Daughters of Bilitis. The name of the organization was taken from an erotic poem by Pierre Louÿs called "Songs of Bilitis." Originally a social club founded to provide a women's alternative to gay bars, the group grew in size and purpose and started publishing a newsletter called *The Ladder*. Primarily collections of poetry, fiction, and biography, *The Ladder* sought to communicate with isolated lesbians. A group of Mattachine Society members published *ONE*, a magazine that dis-

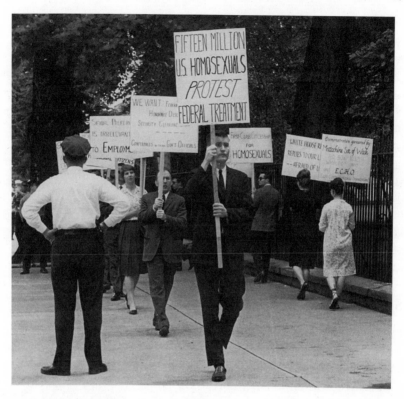

A protest organized by the Mattachine Society in front of the White House,
May 21, 1965. (UPI Telephoto/Bettmann)

cussed theory and political strategy, and later formed ONE, Inc., the
only group whose membership had significant representation of both
genders.

The homophile groups never managed the transition from local
activist groups to national organizations. As the organizations grew,
conflicts over their mission and especially over their tactics dogged
the Mattachine Society, the Daughters of Bilitis, and ONE, Inc.
Membership waxed and waned, focus often wandered, and infighting
among the leadership of the various groups crippled the movement for
years.

Although the homophile organizations fell short of achieving many
of their goals, they nevertheless laid vital groundwork for the next
stage of the homosexual emancipation movement. Several chapters of

the homophile organizations remained active through the 1960s and early 1970s and provided a base for the explosive growth of the movement that would occur after the Stonewall Riots. Homophile periodicals such as *The Ladder*, the *Mattachine Review*, and *Homophile Studies* carried a message of affirmation to the thousands of gays and lesbians who could gain access to them. Most important, the homophile organizations made homosexuality and homosexuals more visible than ever before in American culture. For the countless numbers of gays and lesbians who did not live in the big cities and could not obtain a copy of *The Ladder* or the *Mattachine Review*, coverage in the general media of the court cases the homophile organizations instigated, the press conferences they gave, and the protest marches they staged provided a message of solidarity and empowerment. It was only a matter of time before these decades of hard work would pay off. No one could know that the payoff would come so explosively.

Stonewall

On June 27, 1969, New York City detectives made what started out as a routine vice raid on the Stonewall Inn, a gay bar in the heart of Greenwich Village. As officers released the bar's customers one by one to the street to wait for transport to the police station, a small crowd gathered on the sidewalk outside the bar. One of the bar's patrons, a lesbian, started struggling with her captors and suddenly the crowd turned on the police. "The cops locked themselves in the bar. It was getting vicious. Then someone set fire to the Stonewall. The cops, they just panicked. They had no back-up. They didn't expect any of this retaliation. But they should have. People were very angry for so long. How long can you live in the closet like that?"[10] A parking meter was ripped from the pavement and used by the angry crowd to batter down the locked door of the bar to get at the police. Reinforcements arrived in time to rescue the trapped officers, but they could do little to manage the crowd who now controlled the streets of the Village. Rioting went on far into the night.

The next night saw gays gathering on the streets again, verbally provoking passing police. The situation soon escalated into rock throwing, and fires were set. Before the second night of the riot was over, four hundred police were battling a crowd estimated at more than two thousand homosexuals. "Gay Liberation" had been born. Energized with self-confidence as never before, gay men and women literally took to the streets. "The next day I had to get up to attend some DOB [Daughters of Bilitis] thing," one lesbian participant recalled. "When I got there I found out what had happened at the Stonewall. From lack of sleep and exhaustion I was sort of feverish and I lay on my couch that evening or the next day thinking, 'We've got to do something! We've got to do something! We can't let this thing pass. . . . We should have a march!' "[11]

The riots inspired a new sense of self-respect in the participants. In the July 3, 1969, issue of the *Village Voice*, counterculture (and homosexual) poet Allen Ginsberg observed, "You know, the guys there were so beautiful. They've lost that wounded look that fags all had ten years ago."[12]

Drawing inspiration from the black civil rights movement and the movement protesting the Viet Nam War, the gay liberation movement was aggressive and confrontational at times. At Radio City Music Hall, an organization called the Gay Activist Alliance disrupted a fund-raiser for New York mayor John Lindsay's presidential campaign. Protestors handcuffed themselves to balcony railings, set off sirens, and showered attendees with leaflets protesting police harassment of gays and lesbians. Police raids on gay bars stopped.

Emboldened by their successes in opposing police harassment, gay liberation activists turned their attention to another historical opponent: the psychiatric profession. In 1970, gay activists stormed the annual meeting of the American Psychiatric Association, confronted psychoanalyst Irving Bieber during a panel discussion on homosexuality, and called him a "motherfucker" in front of his shocked colleagues. A wave of protests stimulated sympathetic psychiatrists to call for the deletion of homosexuality from the APA's official list of mental disorders.[13]

After several years of examining the evidence (notably the work of Hooker and Kinsey), a scientific committee of the APA recommended that homosexuality in and of itself no longer be considered a psychiatric illness. The Board of Trustees of the American Psychiatric Association accepted the recommendations of the scientific committee in December 1973, but a small group of psychoanalysts under the leadership of Charles Socarides used a technical ploy to manipulate a membershipwide referendum on the issue. The American Psychiatric Association, which had never previously and has never subsequently settled scientific questions by plebiscite, was forced to do so in the spring of 1974. A clear majority of the membership agreed with the scientific panel and eliminated homosexuality from the third edition of the Diagnostic and Statistical Manual of the Association. Not satisfied, Socarides' group demanded an investigation into the referendum. The APA wearily appointed the Ad Hoc Committee to Investigate the Conduct of the Referendum, which quickly affirmed the results of the vote, declaring that "referenda on facts of science make no sense" and recommending that APA procedures be changed to prevent similar fiascoes in the future. In 1975, homosexual psychiatrists organized themselves, and the Gay, Lesbian, and Bisexual Caucus became an official division of the American Psychiatric Association.

AIDS

In the fall of 1980, doctors were perplexed by reports of an unusually high number of men in their thirties and forties who were falling ill with some very uncommon illnesses: a type of pneumonia caused by the rare microorganism *Pneumocystis carinii*, brain abscesses caused by an animal parasite called toxoplasma, and Kaposi's sarcoma, a rare form of cancer usually seen in the elderly. There were two sets of facts about these unusual cases which suggested that they were connected in some way. One concerned the illnesses: they were all usually seen in individuals who had malfunctioning immune systems. The other concerned the patients: they were all homosexual.

The facts have all come together now: the cause of these illnesses was a virus, eventually named the human immunodeficiency virus (HIV), which slowly destroys the immune system of those infected with it. For a time, the syndrome was called *gay-related immune disorder* (GRID) and was sometimes referred to informally as the "gay plague."[14]

For several years, the media was all but silent about the illness. Aside from articles on the inside pages of a few newspapers, there was little coverage. A "gay-related" disease, after all, affected only a tiny percentage of the population, and discussions of homosexuality were still uncommon in newspapers and all but unknown on television.

Gradually, it became known that HIV infected people regardless of their sexual orientation, and the illness was renamed acquired immune deficiency syndrome, or AIDS. Even before HIV was isolated, several facts about AIDS strongly suggested that it was caused by a virus transmitted through sexual contact or through contact with infected blood. One observation was the striking resemblance of the groups who were coming down with AIDS to the groups known to be at high risk for another viral disease: hepatitis B (sexually promiscuous gay men and intravenous drug users). Despite the emerging evidence that the illness was spread through sexual contact, there was, at first, tremendous resistance on the part of the leaders of some gay organizations to confront this fact and take appropriate action. For some gay men, same-sex eroticism defined not merely their sexual orientation but their identity as individuals. Thus, for them, a gay man who did not have sex whenever, and with whomever, he wanted was denying his true identity; he was repressing his sexuality because of "internalized homophobia." Gay activists demonstrated in some cities to stop public health officials from closing down "bathhouses," sex clubs offering quick and easy anonymous sex with multiple partners. One leader in the San Francisco gay community found himself being called a "sexual Nazi" by other gay men for daring to suggest that they needed to stop visiting bathhouses and rein in promiscuous sexuality.[15]

But while denial, misplaced anger, and hubris blinded some gays to the realities of what was rapidly becoming an epidemic, others, often joined by their lesbian friends and neighbors, mounted a response to it. Gay communities started clinics and other service agencies to provide care for people with AIDS when existing public and private health facilities were still all but ignoring the epidemic. Risk-reduction education programs mounted by gay organizations invented the phrase "safer sex" when public health departments were still trying to come up with ways of educating people about AIDS without talking about sex—especially gay sex.

When a blood test for HIV became available in 1984, the catastrophic dimensions of the epidemic began to emerge. Sixty-five percent of the gay men visiting one venereal disease clinic in San Francisco that year tested positive for the virus.[16] Despite growing numbers of persons infected, sick, or dead from the disease, secrecy and outright denial reigned. In 1985, when actor Rock Hudson collapsed and was taken to a hospital in Paris, a press agent initially gave out the story that he had liver cancer. Only later did the truth emerge that he had come to Paris to be treated at the prestigious Pasteur Institute for AIDS. With the revelation of the truth about Hudson's illness, AIDS became a household word in the United States. Another word also began to appear much more frequently in newspapers and on television: *homosexual*.

The tumultuous conglomeration of social, medical, and political developments affecting homosexuals—especially gay men—which have grown out of the epidemic since the early 1980s is overwhelming; only a few will be mentioned here. For one, the epidemic accelerated a process that had started years before, when riots had broken out in Greenwich Village. The message coming out of the Village's riots and their aftermath had been that homosexuals had much to gain by being visible and demanding better treatment from mainstream society—and much to lose by remaining invisible. But activists had found it difficult to get gay men and lesbians to leave the safety of the gay bars, the nightclubs in the "gay ghettos" of the big cities and resort towns, and show up at demonstrations, hearings, and fund-raising events. With the appearance of AIDS, the appeal to "come out" became more urgent, perhaps crystallized in the message that appeared on placards and tee shirts worn by demonstrators advocating for AIDS-related causes: "Silence = Death." The epidemic mobilized gay and lesbian communities as nothing had before. AIDS also forced American society to begin discussing homosexuality as never before. Tragically, in too many families and too many towns, it took sons and brothers coming home to die to begin the dialogue.

Public health research has indicated that information about AIDS transmission as well as efforts that increase social supports, personal esteem, and positive self-identity reduces the likelihood that gay men will indulge in high-risk sexual practices.[17] It has become even clearer not only that silence equals death but that lack of information about the details of sexuality, isolation from a community of peers, and the self-loathing induced by stigmatization do as well.

AIDS service agencies begun by communities of homosexuals have spurred others in these communities to organize "coming out" groups for individuals coming to terms with homosexuality, support groups for adolescents struggling with sexual orientation identity issues, and substance abuse programs targeting gays and lesbians. Homosexuality is not just about sex, and neither is AIDS prevention: it's also about self-acceptance, destigmatization, and tolerance.

Beyond Stonewall

By the late 1980s, so many gays and lesbians had insisted on visibility for so long that strict enforcement of crimes-against-nature statutes became almost impossible. The pace of emancipation accelerated, and soon such laws were being repealed across the country and civil rights statutes broadened to include "sexual orientation" as a protected status in several cities, and then several states. Hundreds of thousands marched in front of the White House in 1993 to call attention to the inequalities still suffered by gay people.

These changes have meant that gay bars are far from the only gay "institution" any more. Professional, civic, and arts associations and organizations have become too numerous to count—from the Gay and Lesbian Medical Association to the Gay and Lesbian Association of Choruses to Digital Queers, a gay computer professionals organization.

Gay and lesbian individuals have not only demanded freedom from threats of imprisonment or being fired from their jobs but increasingly have insisted on recognition and sanction of their relationships. In 1991, the software giant Lotus Development Corporation began offering partners of gay and lesbian employees the same benefits package available to the spouses of its married workers, the first "Fortune 500" company to do so. Many others have followed suit, including, in 1995, the Walt Disney Company (despite receiving a warning from fifteen Florida state legislators that to do so would be "a big mistake both morally and financially").[18] On August 1, 1994, Vermont was the first of the fifty states to offer domestic partnership benefits to all state employees.

The pace of these victories continues to accelerate with too many recent landmark events to list. Those struggling with sexual orientation issues in their lives no longer need struggle alone and be confronted with unremittingly negative images of homosexuals. Hundreds of little steps bring gay and lesbian people further into the mainstream of society. Movie and television screens are increasingly populated with accurately portrayed gay and lesbian characters instead of negative stereotypes. Car rental companies and health clubs extend "couples' rates" to same-sex couples. In 1994, Britain's BBC extended "honeymoon leave" benefits to gay and lesbian employees, entitling them to an additional week off from work and a gift certificate of £75 (about $112). New Jersey governor Christine Todd Whitman proclaimed the week of October 8, 1994, as "National Coming-Out Week" in New Jersey, four months after she had proclaimed "Lesbian, Bisexual, and Gay Pride Month" to mark the twenty-fifth anniversary of the Stonewall Riots.

Today gay and lesbian Americans find themselves in a more friendly world, but still a world that is characterized by conflict and contradictions. For example, Duke University extended its employee benefits package to partners of gay and lesbian employees in 1995, even though laws that punish private homosexual acts between consenting adults with prison terms are on the books in the university's home state of North Carolina. Sodomy laws, antidiscrimination laws and policies, marriage and adoption laws, and policies involving gay membership in the military continue to be debated in the courts and on ballots all over the country. Although complete recognition and acceptance of homosexual persons as equals everywhere in our society has not yet arrived, more gays and lesbians than ever before are "coming out," speaking out, and getting involved, empowering themselves and their supporters to make their futures better. The road to emancipation has never been clearer—and never have so many walked it.

Summing Up

Unanswered Questions

Many people have questions about homosexuality which they ask for many reasons. I wrote this book for those who are looking for information to better understand themselves, or their children, or their friends, co-workers, students, parishioners, neighbors. It's not really possible to understand the complex and subtle answers to these questions unless one understands some key facts about homosexuality. Without these facts, making sense out of news stories about "gay genes," conflicts over sexuality education in schools, AIDS prevention, civil rights legislation for homosexuals, and so on becomes an elusive quest. I've tried to convey the essential facts to you, but I hope I've done more. I hope I've persuaded you that understanding homosexuality requires thoughtful analysis from several different perspectives: historical, biological, psychological, and political. The answers to most questions about homosexuality are incomplete unless all the different perspectives are included. This book cannot—no book can—answer all the questions, but if this volume has laid some factual groundwork and given you new perspectives to explore, then I've accomplished my goal.

We have covered a lot of ground in this attempt to understand homosexuality better—from ancient Greece to the Knights Templar to the Stonewall Inn, neurons, hormones, and chromosomes, left hand, right brain, the Rorschach test, the Kinsey scale, nature and nurture, "coming out," and Digital Queers—and we've only scratched the surface. A whole book could be devoted to nearly every topic we've covered—from sexual anthropology to zygotes. And I've left a lot of questions unanswered.

"Sexual Histories" focused almost exclusively on northern European and American history and sociology. What about other societies? What effect has the greater dominance of the Catholic Church and the culture of machismo had on attitudes toward homosexuality in southern European countries? Spain burned more homosexuals at the stake than any other European country during the Middle Ages, but some of the kingdoms of Italy were among the least repressive medieval states. How can this contrast be explained? A complete cultural survey would have examined homosexuality in ancient Persia and the effect of the rise of Islam on homosexuality in the modern Middle East, the transsexual castes of India, the "Passion of the Cut Sleeve" in China,[1] and many, many other cultures and customs.

The subtleties of sexual biology would literally take a lifetime to explore completely—scientists have spent entire careers seeking to understand a single hormone or brain center. As more and more sophisticated probes into the workings of the cell are developed, we will learn more and more about the biology of sexual orientation in the years to come. This area of knowledge will undoubtedly provide the richest source of completely new information about homosexuality—and, perhaps, the most troublesome. If and when specific genes linked to homosexuality are discovered, what are the ethics of testing for these genes in fetuses? In adults?

Sexual identities and homosexual identity developmental models continue to change. Will models for understanding sexual orientation development today be valid in ten years? In five years? How is the process different for men and women? For adolescents in urban versus rural areas? For African American versus white versus Latino versus any other ethnic group you care to consider? What about economic factors? What is the effect of homosexuality on the family members who are not homosexual? When I attended a conference sponsored by the organization Parents and Family and Friends of Lesbians and Gays (P-FLAG), I heard parents of homosexual children talk about their own "coming out" process—acknowledging to others that their child is gay or lesbian—a process I frankly hadn't really ever thought about. What are the steps in the parents' "coming out"? The siblings'? Sexual politics promises to be with us for a long time to come. The courts still have not answered some very basic questions on the issue of homosexuality: Are homosexuals a minority? Are certain legal privileges and protections, like marriage, meant to be enjoyed by heterosexuals only? Is it right to give exemptions from nondiscrimination laws to religious groups and allow them to exclude homosexuals as employees? Would it be legal to exclude a student from a religious college who announced she or he was gay? The conflicts over the role and rights of homosexuals in the military continue to fester. More than seventeen thousand individuals were separated from the United States military because of homosexuality between 1980 and 1990, individuals who had cost taxpayers perhaps five hundred million dollars to recruit and train.[2] Is this expense, and the emotional impact on the gay and lesbian individuals forced out, justified?

Conclusions

It may be argued that "homosexuals" didn't exist until about 150 years ago. Homosexuality certainly did, as our historical survey showed, but individuals who fell in love with members of their own sex weren't thought to be a particular kind of person. Some societies, such as classical Greece, didn't feel the need to label the phenomenon and had no words for homosexuality. Same-sex eroticism was something a few individuals seemed to prefer more than their fellows, but it wasn't thought to be a characteristic worth inventing a name for. Often, the gender of one's sexual partners was less important than attributes like their age and social status. This being the case, homosexuality was in a sense "submerged" within these cultures—attracting no special notice. On the other hand, some societies, such as many in pre-Columbian America, recognized a separate class of persons whose gender and sexual orientation was different and afforded them a special status. Sometimes this special status was a favored one, sometimes not. In times and cultures in which individual behavior was highly regulated in deference to group solidarity, such as among the ancient Aztecs and Israelites, reproductive sexuality was the mandate and any other form of sexual expression forbidden and punished.

Although same-sex eroticism is interesting, a pleasant diversion, or an acceptable substitute for many, it is an urgent and compelling sexuality for only a comparatively small minority. Thus, homosexuality has become easily associated with the outsider, the different, the unfamiliar. The study of the forces of stigma and bigotry shows us that "unfamiliar" to "dangerous" is a step easily taken among humans. Homosexuals in Western society have been identified with others considered dangerous persons since the late Middle Ages: sinners, infidels, foreign enemies, heretics, the mentally ill, political subversives, race defilers, criminals.

For several hundreds of years, the institutions of the majority considered homosexuality something a person *did* and called it sodomy, buggery, or a crime against nature. During the nineteenth century, a conceptual shift occurred, and a few individuals began to talk about homosexuality as something a person *was*. A new vocabulary was invented for these persons: Urning, invert—homosexual.

The sciences of behavior began to explore human sexual behavior but could not shake loose the dread of the sexually different inherited from the institution whose authority science was supplanting: the church. Without examining the validity of their premise, behavioral scientists looked for the pathology they assumed to underlie this "illness." Finding none in the body, medicine turned to psychoanalysis, a new method of investigation into the basis of human behavior which claimed to have a unique ability to see into the mind. Confused and murky circular reasoning derived from an arcane system of symbolism and interpretation was applied to cases of unhappy, even emotionally disturbed, homosexuals to justify "treatment" of their "condition." No one thought to look for happy and healthy homosexuals to understand homosexuality because psychoanalytic theory declared that there were no such creatures. The invert is homosexual because he is psychologically disturbed. How do we know this? Because the inverts who come to us to be cured of their homosexuality tell us so.

In the late twentieth century, the sciences of biology have again begun to consider the phenomenon of homosexuality and to apply techniques and develop theories to understand it which depend on verifiable measurements. In measuring the size of certain brain structures, performance on psychological tests, and the structure of chromosomes, differences are found between homosexual and heterosexual individuals—*differences*, not abnormalities. The emerging science of the mind, which springs from knowledge of the biology of the brain, proposes that the developing mind molds itself to the world in which it finds itself. Language, cooperation—culture—require that the brain be full of potentialities and free to develop in many directions. A society of human creatures too rigidly programmed for reproductive behavior would not be very human.

The preponderance of the scientific evidence is converging on a view that homosexual people have had of themselves for as long as any had the courage to record it. Homosexuality is a natural, abiding, normal sexuality for some people. It is not a disease state, not simply a behavior, and not subject to change. It develops in some individuals as a result of influences of heredity, prenatal development, childhood experiences, and cultural milieu in varying combinations. No one influence seems either necessary or sufficient—homosexual orientation is a possible outcome in many different circumstances because the human mind is uniquely evolved to be rich in possibilities.

Fear of homosexuals has been exploited by the unscrupulous and the misguided in the pursuit of wealth, power, revenge, political influence, and cultural control. Long linked with other dangerous outsiders in the minds of those alarmed by human differences, homosexuals have been marginalized, persecuted, exiled, and imprisoned, hunted down and murdered.

The deeply ingrained antipathy toward homosexuals and the frightening consequences of being identified as homosexual have meant that people identifying homosexual feelings within themselves often experience a crisis of identity. Some weather the storm, some unfortunately perish, and many carry the emotional scars of stigmatization for many years. Some hate what they are and seek to "heal" themselves. Misguided and unscrupulous counselors accept them into a conspiracy of fear and loathing, preaching redemption and teaching self-hatred, practicing brainwashing and calling it "reparative therapy."

Gay and lesbian people first demanded the right to be left alone and then, more recently, the right to be included—their love and relationships accepted and validated. It is possible that prejudice against homosexuals will one day be as unacceptable in our society as prejudice against ethnic or religious minorities—and perceived as just as irrational. Much progress has been made, but much work remains. For a hundred years or so, gay and lesbian people have struggled against forces that would oppress and persecute them. Some of them were given a pink triangle to wear and were murdered for their protest. Many more now proudly put on a pink triangle and march down Main Street to celebrate who they are. They march for acceptance and freedom and call on their family and friends to join them.

Yet, Freedom! yet thy banner, torn, but flying,
Streams like the thunderstorm *against* the wind.
—Lord Byron

Notes

CHAPTER ONE Before Homosexuality

1. Margaret Mead, *Sex and Temperament in Three Primitive Societies* (New York: Morrow, 1935), v.

2. E. M. Forster, *Maurice* (New York: Norton, 1971), 51.

3. Plato, *Charmides*, quoted in Kenneth J. Dover, *Greek Homosexuality* (Cambridge: Harvard University Press, 1978).

4. Plato, *Symposium*, in *Great Dialogues of Plato*, ed. Eric Warmington and Phillip Rouse (New York: New American Library, 1984), 85–87.

5. Euripides, *The Cyclops*, quoted in David F. Greenberg, *The Construction of Homosexuality* (Chicago: University of Chicago Press, 1988), 145.

6. David Halperin, "One Hundred Years of Homosexuality," *Diacritics* (Summer 1986): 39.

7. David Halperin, *One Hundred Years of Homosexuality* (New York: Routledge, 1990), 90.

8. Plato, *Symposium*, 82.

9. Greenberg, *Construction of Homosexuality*, 145.

10. Plato, *Symposium*, 88.

11. David Halperin, "Homosexuality," in *The Oxford Classical Dictionary*, 3d ed. (New York: Oxford University Press, in press).

12. Ibid.

13. Dolores Klaich, *Woman plus Woman* (Tallahassee: Naiad Press, 1989; reprint of *Woman + Woman*, New York: Morrow, 1974).

14. Most of the information in this section is taken from Walter Williams, *The*

Spirit and the Flesh: Sexual Diversity in American Indian Culture (Boston: Beacon Press, 1988), an excellent source of information on the berdache.

15. Greenberg, *Construction of Homosexuality*, 41.

16. Neil Miller, *Out of the Past: Gay and Lesbian History from 1869 to the Present* (New York: Vintage Press, 1995), 37.

17. Quoted in ibid., 35.

18. See Ruth Underhill, *Social Organization of the Papago Indians* (New York: Columbia University Press, 1938).

19. Williams, *Spirit and the Flesh*, 19.

20. Ibid., 24–26.

21. Jonathan Ned Katz, *Gay American History* (New York: Thomas Y. Crowell, 1976), 310.

22. Greenberg, *Construction of Homosexuality*, 166.

23. In his original writings, Herdt used pseudonyms for the real places where the "Sambia" (also a pseudonym) live. Herdt promised his subjects that he would disguise their identity and the location of their homeland in all his writings to protect the secrecy of their rituals. A good introduction to this work is Gilbert Herdt, *Guardians of the Flutes, Idioms of Masculinity* (New York: Columbia University Press, 1987). As the Sambia have become more assimilated into modern Papua New Guinea, they have abandoned these rituals.

24. John Money, *Gay, Straight, and In-between: The Sexology of Erotic Orientation* (New York: Oxford University Press, 1988).

25. Herdt, *Guardians of the Flutes*, 282.

26. Ibid., 252 n.

CHAPTER TWO   **Sodomites and Urnings**

1. David F. Greenberg, *The Construction of Homosexuality* (Chicago: University of Chicago Press, 1988), 227.

2. The complexities of scriptural interpretation being beyond the scope of this book, not to mention the ken of this author, I have consciously (though perhaps pusillanimously) avoided a detailed discussion of the Scriptures and the writings of the early church fathers, including Saint Paul. For a superb explication of the scriptural references interpreted by medieval theologians to form a basis for the Christian condemnation of homosexuality, see John Boswell, *Christianity, Social Tolerance, and Homosexuality: Gay People in Western Europe from the Beginning of the Christian Era to the Fourteenth Century* (Chicago: University of Chicago Press, 1980). This book, as well as John J. McNeill, *The Church and the Homosexual* (Boston: Beacon Press, 1988), convincingly makes the point that the Bible does not condemn all homosexual acts and that Christian condemnation of homosexuality developed during the late Middle Ages in response to political and social upheavals across Europe. See especially chap. 10 in Boswell and also chap. 7 in Greenberg, *Construction of Homosexuality*.

3. Boswell, *Christianity, Social Tolerance, and Homosexuality*, 243.

4. Greenberg, *Construction of Homosexuality*, 259. See also Boswell, *Christianity, Social Tolerance, and Homosexuality*, 287–88.

5. Boswell, *Christianity, Social Tolerance, and Homosexuality*, 277.

6. Quoted and translated in ibid., 231.

7. Hubert Kennedy, *Ulrichs: The Life and Works of Karl Heinrich Ulrichs* (Boston: Alyson, 1988), 19.

8. These works have now been translated into English as Karl Heinrich Ulrichs, *The Riddle of "Man-manly Love": The Pioneering Work on Male Homosexuality* [Forschungen über das Rätsel der Mannmännlichen Lieben], trans. Michael A. Lombardi-Nash (Buffalo: Prometheus, 1994).

9. Quoted in Kennedy, *Ulrichs*, 50.

10. King Ludwig II of Bavaria was another homosexual king deposed by his government. In 1886, Ludwig was arrested by a parliamentary commission at his almost completed fairy-tale castle, Neuschwanstein. Within forty-eight hours, he was dead, drowned in Starnberg Lake on the grounds of the castle which had been prepared for his house arrest. Whether he was a victim of suicide or assassination has never been established.

11. Kennedy, *Ulrichs*, 109.

12. Quoted in ibid., 71.

13. Richard von Krafft-Ebing, *Psychopathia Sexualis*, trans. Franklin Klaf (New York: Bell, 1965), 295.

CHAPTER THREE   Perversion and Inversion

1. Havelock Ellis and John Addington Symonds, *Sexual Inversion* (London, 1897; reprint, New York: Arno Press, 1975).

2. Richard von Krafft-Ebing, *Psychopathia Sexualis*, trans. Franklin Klaf (New York: Bell, 1965), 255, 232, 245, 281.

3. Ibid., 190.

4. Ibid., 190–93.

5. Ibid., 223.

6. As originally described in a letter from Brown to the librarian dated December 21, 1925, quoted in *The Memoirs of John Addington Symonds*, ed. Phyllis Grosskurth (New York: Random House, 1984).

7. *Memoirs of John Addington Symonds*, 11.

8. Ibid., 182; written in May 1889.

9. Ibid., 85.

10. Ibid., 73.

11. Ibid., 94–96.

12. Ibid., 99.

13. Ibid., 104.

14. Ibid., 124–25.

15. Ibid., 128.

16. Ibid., 152.

17. Ibid., 157.

18. Ibid., 184–85.

19. Symonds, "A Problem in Greek Ethics," appendix 1 in Ellis and Symonds, *Sexual Inversion.*

20. See Richard Ellman, *Oscar Wilde* (New York: Alfred A. Knopf, 1987), 409 n.

21. Hubert Kennedy, *Ulrichs: The Life and Works of Karl Heinrich Ulrichs* (Boston: Alyson, 1988), 218.

22. Phyllis Grosskurth, *Havelock Ellis: A Biography* (New York: Alfred A. Knopf, 1980), 186–87.

23. Ibid., 194. The Bedborough incident was not the last of the scandals to swirl around *Sexual Inversion.* In 1899, Ellis learned that the publishing house that had produced the first editions of the book was a money-laundering operation run by a German with the fantastic name of George Ferdinand Springmühl von Weissenfeld. Von Weissenfeld had amassed a fortune from various fraudulent schemes by the time the police caught up with him in a Cambridge mansion complete with secret doors and hidden passages. As he was being arrested, von Weissenfeld took poison hidden in his ring and dropped dead on the spot.

24. Ellis and Symonds, *Sexual Inversion*, 92–93, 46–47.

25. Ibid., 68.

26. John Addington Symonds, *Male Love: A Problem in Greek Ethics and Other Writings*, ed. Robert Peters (New York: Pagan Press, 1983), 149.

27. Ellis and Symonds, *Sexual Inversion*, 137.

28. Ellis would return to this theme in later volumes of *Studies in the Psychology of Sex.* He was one of the first medical writers to question the validity of "masturbatory insanity." The Victorians had a singular horror of masturbation (which they called "onanism" after Onan, son of Judah in Genesis, who displeased God by "spill[ing] his semen on the ground" (Gen. 38:9). The White Cross League was one of several "moral purity" organizations that sprang up during the Victorian era to advocate sexual continence and publicize the terrible consequences of "self-abuse," thought to range from impotence to psychosis. A full discussion of the moral purity movement is contained in Lesley Hall, "Forbidden by God, Despised by Men: Masturbation, Medical Warnings, Moral Panic, and Manhood in Great Britain, 1850–1950," in *Forbidden History: The State, Society, and the Regulation of Sexuality in Modern Europe*, ed. John Fout (Chicago: University of Chicago Press, 1992).

29. Ellis and Symonds, *Sexual Inversion*, 107.

30. Ibid., 110. Ellis postulated "a congenital abnormality" to explain homosexuality but admitted he did not know where to look for such an abnormality. He specifically rejected Ulrichs' idea of *anima maliebris in corpore virili inclusa.* (Symonds, though otherwise impressed by Ulrichs' ideas, dismissed "the hypothesis

of a female soul shut up within a male body" as "bygone scholastic speculation" [*Memoirs of John Addington Symonds*, 64].) Ellis was no more impressed with the biologically flavored concept "that in inversion a female brain is combined with a male body or male glands. This is . . . not explanation. It merely crystallizes into an epigram the superficial impression of the matter. . . . To assert that a female soul or even a female brain is expressing itself through a male body . . . is simply unintelligible." Ellis and Symonds, *Sexual Inversion*, 131–32.

31. Ellis and Symonds, *Sexual Inversion*, 132, 134.

32. Ellis did, however, believe that the prevention of homosexuality might be possible and to that end advocated "co-education of the sexes," presumably to lessen the incidence of the "schoolboy homosexuality" Symonds had noted. (Whether an increase in the incidence of boy-girl sexual contact was the hoped-for result of coeducation is not specified.)

33. Ellis and Symonds, *Sexual Inversion*, 146.

34. In his splendid biography of Victoria, Stanley Weintraub recounts a vivid though apocryphal account of Victoria's reaction to the Labouchèe Criminal Law Amendment making "gross indecencies" between men a crime. When the bill was presented to the queen for her signature, she read the provision recognizing the existence of homosexual behavior between females. She reportedly questioned the need for the section, saying, "Women don't do such things." Rather than explain otherwise, her ministers changed the law to omit references to lesbianism. See Stanley Weintraub, *Victoria: An Intimate Biography* (New York: Truman Talley Books, 1987).

35. Ellis and Symonds, *Sexual Inversion*, 147.

CHAPTER FOUR   Women's Voices

1. John Boswell, *Christianity, Social Tolerance, and Homosexuality: Gay People in Western Europe from the Beginning of the Christian Era to the Fourteenth Century* (Chicago: University of Chicago Press, 1980), 158.

2. Quoted in ibid., 220.

3. Quoted in Rose Collins, *Portraits to the Wall: Historic Lesbian Lives Unveiled* (London: Cassell, 1994), 16.

4. Ibid., 17.

5. Ibid.

6. After John Churchill died in 1722, Sarah Churchill dismissed the architect he had hired and supervised the construction herself. She did the same at their London home, Marlborough House (also a gift from Anne), this time sacking no less an architect than Sir Christopher Wren.

7. One such song went:

When as Queen Anne of great renown
Great Britain's Scepter sway'd

Besides the Church, she dearly lov'd
A dirty chambermaid.

Her secretary, she was not,
Because she could not write,
But had the Conduct and the Care
Of some dark Deeds at Night.

Quoted in Collins, *Portraits to the Wall.*

8. After Anne's death, Sarah made yet another and perhaps even more brazen attempt to link her family to the Crown. She offered Anne's cousin, the Prince of Wales, one hundred thousand pounds to marry her granddaughter—a young woman by the name of Lady Diana Spencer (an ancestor of the current wife of the modern Prince Charles).

9. Helena Whitbread, *I Know My Own Heart: The Diaries of Anne Lister, 1791–1840* (New York: New York University Press, 1988) and *No Priest but Love: Excerpts from the Diaries of Anne Lister, 1824–1826* (New York: New York University Press, 1992).

10. Whitbread, *I Know My Own Heart*, xxiv.

11. Ibid., 5.

12. Ibid., 8.

13. Ibid.

14. Ibid., 145.

15. Ibid., 262.

16. Whitbread, *No Priest but Love*, 47.

17. Ibid., 49.

18. Ibid., 151.

19. Ibid., 153.

20. Ruth Perry, "Colonizing the Breast: Sexuality and Maternity in Eighteenth Century England," in *Forbidden History: The State, Society, and the Regulation of Sexuality in Modern Europe*, ed. John Fout (Chicago: University of Chicago Press, 1992).

21. Lillian Faderman's book on women's friendships, *Surpassing the Love of Men: Romantic Friendship and Love between Women from the Renaissance to the Present* (New York: Quill, 1981), cannot be too highly recommended.

22. Quoted in ibid., 176.

23. Ibid., 120–25.

24. Whitbread, *I Know My Own Heart*, 210.

25. Faderman, *Surpassing the Love of Men*, 26.

26. Ibid., 451.

27. Quoted in Lillian Faderman, *Odd Girls and Twilight Lovers: A History of Lesbian Life in Twentieth Century America* (New York: Penguin, 1991), 31.

28. The Women's Fund Committee also commissioned John Singer Sargent to

paint a portrait of Mary Garrett for the university. The portrait still occupies a place of honor in the ornate reading room of the medical school's library.

29. Faderman, *Surpassing the Love of Men*, 190.

30. Ibid., 168.

31. Ibid., 191.

32. Ibid., 147–52. American playwright Lillian Hellman based her play *The Children's Hour* on the trial.

33. Carroll Smith-Rosenberg, "Discourses of Sexuality and Subjectivity: The New Women, 1870–1936," in *Hidden from History: Reclaiming the Gay and Lesbian Past*, ed. Martin Duberman, Martha Vicinus, and George Chauncey Jr. (New York: New American Library, 1989).

34. Richard von Krafft-Ebing, *Psychopathia Sexualis*, trans. Franklin Klaf (New York: Bell, 1965), 263.

35. Irving D. Steinhardt, *Ten Sex Talks with Girls* (1914), quoted in Faderman, *Odd Girls and Twilight Lovers*, 37.

36. Quoted in Ester Newton, "The Mythic Mannish Lesbian: Radclyffe Hall and the New Woman," in Duberman, Vicinus, and Chauncey, *Hidden from History*, 286.

37. Quoted in George Chauncey Jr., "From Sexual Inversion to Homosexuality: Medicine and the Changing Conceptualization of Female Deviance," *Salmagundi* 58–59 (1982–83): 114–45.

38. R. W. Shufedt in the *Pacific Medical Journal* (1902), quoted in Smith-Rosenberg, "Discourses of Sexuality," 271.

39. James Weir Jr., "The Effects of Female Suffrage on Posterity," *American Naturalist* 24, no. 345 (September 1895): 815–25, quoted in Faderman, *Odd Girls and Twilight Lovers*, 46.

40. See Faderman, *Surpassing the Love of Men*, 392–406.

41. Quoted in Dolores Klaich, *Woman plus Woman* (Tallahassee: Naiad Press, 1989; reprint of *Woman + Woman*, New York: Morrow, 1974), 194.

42. Quoted in ibid., 186.

43. Ibid., 184.

44. Quoted in Faderman, *Surpassing the Love of Men*, 321.

CHAPTER FIVE   **Psychoanalysis**

1. The ancient Greeks had also recognized these mysterious ailments, which seemed especially common in women, and postulated that they were related to sexual functioning—specifically to childlessness and sexual abstinence. Believing that the empty womb somehow caused the symptoms, the Greeks called the problem "hysteria" after the Greek word for "uterus."

2. In a short history of psychoanalysis written in 1914, Freud credited Charcot with being one of the originators of this idea. Although Charcot, like his contemporaries, taught that some unknown nervous system degeneration caused hysteri-

cal symptoms, he had another theory that he didn't mention in any of his lectures. Freud learned of this other theory at a reception one evening when he overheard Charcot saying to another physician: "Dans des cas pareils, c'est toujours la chose genital, toujours . . . toujours" [In these cases, it's always a sexual thing, always . . . always]. Freud was "almost paralysed with amazement" and said to himself: "Well, but if he knows that, why does he never say so?" See Sigmund Freud, "On the History of the Psychoanalytic Movement," in *The Standard Edition of the Complete Psychological Works of Sigmund Freud*, vol. 14, ed. and trans. James Strachey (London: Hogarth, 1957), 14.

3. Quoted in Kenneth Lewes, *The Psychoanalytic Theory of Male Homosexuality* (New York: Simon and Schuster, 1988), 35.

4. Ibid.

5. Sigmund Freud, "Three Essays on the Theory of Sexuality," in *Standard Edition*, vol. 7:123.

6. Sigmund Freud, "Analysis of a Phobia in a Five Year Old Boy" (1909), in *Standard Edition*, vol. 10, 1–147.

7. Sigmund Freud, "Certain Neurotic Mechanisms in Jealousy, Paranoia, and Homosexuality" (1922), in *Standard Edition*, vol. 18, 221–34.

8. Sigmund Freud, "The Psychogenesis of a Case of Homosexuality in a Woman" (1920), in *Standard Edition*, vol. 18, 155–72.

9. Psychoanalysis has been said to employ *hermeneutic* reasoning. Hermeneutics is the study of methods of interpretation, and the term usually refers to the study of interpretation of religious scriptures. Like the interpretation of scripture, psychoanalytic interpretation requires that the interpreter believe in a system of meanings and symbols that are not apparent in the "text"—in this case, the conscious mind of the analysand. As one contemporary psychiatric text puts it, the psychoanalyst "seeks in the text of consciousness, the underlying meanings he knows are there." See Paul McHugh and Phillip Slavney, *The Perspectives of Psychiatry* (Baltimore: Johns Hopkins University Press, 1986), 20.

10. Sigmund Freud, "On the History of the Psychoanalytic Movement" (1914), *Standard Edition*, vol. 14, 34 n.

11. At least some of this distortion derives from the work of James Strachey, who translated Freud's works into English. For example, it was Strachey who invented the words *ego, id, cathexis,* and so forth. In the original German works, Freud used ordinary German words to label these concepts. For example, Freud's "*Das Ich*" ("the I") became "the Ego" in the standard English translation. This and other translation problems have been said to have the effect of hardening Freud's more humanistic and philosophical style of reasoning and making his ideas sound more rigid and "scientific" than Freud meant them to be. See Darius Ornston, "Strachey's Influence," *International Journal of Psychoanalysis* 63 (1982): 409–25.

12. Sigmund Freud, "Letter to an American Mother" (1935), published in *American Journal of Psychiatry* 107 (1951): 786.

13. Freud, "Case of Homosexuality in a Woman," 169.

14. See Lewes, *Psychoanalytic Theory*, for a complete discussion of the development of these ideas.

15. Edmund Bergler, *Homosexuality: Disease or Way of Life?* (New York: Hill and Wang, 1956), 9.

16. Lewes, *Psychoanalytic Theory*, 32.

17. Bergler, *Homosexuality*, 8.

18. This is not to say that all psychoanalytic clinicians still believe that homosexuality is pathological. In *Being Homosexual: Gay Men and Their Development* (New York: Farrar, Straus & Giroux, 1989), Richard Isay describes psychoanalytic therapy with gay men in whom homosexuality is regarded as normal and healthy for them. Other psychoanalysts have written that "[psycho-]analysis of homosexuality in terms of psychic conflicts is 'outdated'" (Michael J. Hurewitz, "Male Homosexuality: A Contemporary Psychoanalytic Perspective," *American Journal of Psychoanalysis* 52, no. 3 [1992]: 294–98) and that "psychoanalytic treatment of [homosexuals] should focus more on the nature of the [patient's] distress, rather than on the fact of homosexuality" (Edwin Wood, "Evolutions of an Orientation Concerning the Nature of the Male Homosexualities," *American Journal of Psychoanalysis* 55, no. 2 [1995]: 103–21).

A recent study, however, demonstrated continuing problems with antihomosexual bias in psychoanalytically trained therapists. Psychoanalytic clinicians presented with a series of nearly identical clinical scenarios tended to make more pathological diagnoses when the patient was identified as gay in the scenario as compared with when the patient was identified as heterosexual. Arthur H. Lilling and Richard Friedman, "Bias towards Gay Patients by Psychoanalytic Clinicians: An Empirical Investigation," *Archives of Sexual Behavior* 24, no. 5 (October 1995): 563–70.

CHAPTER SIX   Surveys and Inkblots

1. Alfred Kinsey, Wardell Pomeroy, and Clyde Martin, *Sexual Behavior in the Human Male* (Philadelphia: W. B. Saunders, 1948), 9.

2. Ibid., 3.

3. Quoted in Wardell Pomeroy, *Dr. Kinsey and the Institute for Sex Research* (New York: Harper & Row, 1972), 245.

4. Pomeroy, *Dr. Kinsey*, 275.

5. Kinsey, *Male*, 625.

6. Ibid., 659.

7. Ibid., 663.

8. Ibid., 651.

9. Ibid., 664.

10. Alfred Kinsey, Wardell Pomeroy, Clyde Martin, and Paul Gebhard, *Sexual Behavior in the Human Female* (Philadelphia: W. B. Saunders, 1953).

11. Ibid., 453.

12. Ibid., 472.

13. Ibid., 469.

14. Edward O. Lauman, John H. Gagnon, Robert T. Michael, and Stuart Michaels, *The Social Organization of Sexuality: Sexual Practices in the United States* (Chicago: University of Chicago Press, 1994).

15. Evelyn Hooker, "The Adjustment of the Male Overt Homosexual," *Journal of Projective Techniques* 21 (1957): 18–31.

16. Ibid., 20.

17. Irving Bieber et al., *Homosexuality: A Psychoanalytic Study of Male Homosexuals* (New York: Basic Books, 1962).

PART TWO   **Sexual Biology**

1. *Newsweek*, February 24, 1992.

2. Paul McHugh and Phillip Slavney, *The Perspectives of Psychiatry* (Baltimore: Johns Hopkins University Press, 1986), 112.

3. John Boswell, "Sexual and Ethical Categories in Pre-modern Europe," in *Homosexuality/Heterosexuality: Concepts of Sexual Orientation*, ed. David Mc-Whirter, Stephanie Sanders, and June Reinisch (New York: Oxford University Press, 1990), 15.

CHAPTER SEVEN   **Sexual Biology I**

1. See Hubert Kennedy, *Ulrichs: The Life and Works of Karl Heinrich Ulrichs* (Boston: Alyson, 1988), 52.

2. Ibid.

3. Havelock Ellis and John Addington Symonds, *Sexual Inversion* (London, 1897; reprint, New York: Arno Press, 1975), 133.

4. See Chapter 5.

5. Female development occurs without any need for hormones secreted by the ovaries; female animal embryos from which the ovaries have been experimentally removed still develop into females. It is only after puberty that high levels of estrogens from the ovaries are necessary for reproduction.

6. Congenital adrenal hyperplasia, the androgen insensitivity syndrome, and other syndromes of sexual misdevelopment due to hormonal and genetic problems are reviewed in Professor John Money's book: *Gay, Straight, and In-between: The Sexology of Erotic Orientation* (New York: Oxford University Press, 1988).

7. A. Ehrhardt et al., "Sexual Orientation after Prenatal Exposure to Exogenous Estrogen," *Archives of Sexual Behavior* 14 (1985): 57–77.

8. Simon LeVay, *The Sexual Brain* (Cambridge: MIT Press, 1993), 134.

9. For a comprehensive scientific overview of the research on rat sexual behaviors and brain structures and their experimental manipulation with hormones, the interested reader is referred to Arnold Gerall, Howard Moltz, and Ingeborg Ward, eds., *Sexual Differentiation*, vol. 11 of *Handbook of Behavioral Neurobiology*, (New York: Plenum Press, 1992).

10. What about the observation that the male rats castrated at birth showed *female* mating behavior if they were injected with testosterone as adults? This apparent contradiction is explained by two further facts. First, during adulthood, testosterone turns out to have an "activating effect" on whatever sexual circuitry is in place, male *or* female Second, the absence of testosterone during the critical period causes a female pattern to emerge. Testosterone during the critical period *organizes* the circuitry for mounting behavior; with no testosterone, the circuitry for lordosis develops. After puberty, testosterone can *activate* mating behaviors of either type, determined by which circuitry is present.

11. L. Allen, M. Hines, J. Shryne, and R. Gorski, "Two Sexually Dimorphic Cell Groups in the Human Brain," *Journal of Neuroscience* 9 (1989): 497–506.

12. Alan Bell, Martin Weinberg, and Sue Hammersmith, *Sexual Preference: Its Development in Men and Women* (Bloomington: Indiana University Press, 1981).

13. Richard Green, "Gender Identity in Childhood and Later Sexual Orientation," *American Journal of Psychiatry* 142 (1985): 339–41.

14. R. Schiavi, A. Theilgaard, D.Owen, and D. White, "Sex Chromosome Anomalies, Hormones, and Sexuality," *Archives of General Psychiatry* 45 (1988): 19–24.

15. June Reinisch and Stephanie Sanders, "Prenatal Hormonal Contributions to Sex Differences in Human Cognitive and Personality Development," in Gerall, Moltz, and Ward, *Sexual Differentiation*, 221–43.

CHAPTER EIGHT   **Sexual Biology II**

1. Norman Geschwind and Albert Galaburda, "Cerebral Lateralization, Biological Mechanisms, Associations, and Pathology II: A Hypothesis and a Program for Research," *Archives of Neurology* 42 (1985): 521–49.

2. Not only does this area organize the intricate and complex muscle movements of the tongue, lips, and larynx necessary for speech, but it also organizes the mental aspect of language, the translation of ideas into words. Some stroke patients with very discrete damage to this speech area have a specific defect of language called *aphasia* (literally "no speech") in which they retain the mechanics of speech but lose the ability to express ideas or name objects.

3. In this section, many comparisons of psychological functioning will be made between men and women and between gay men and lesbians and their nongay counterparts. It is important to remember that statements about the "superiority" of one group over another in a particular area is true for *average* levels of functioning only. Although a group of men may perform better on average than a group of

women on a particular task, there are often some women who perform *better* than most men on that same task. This wide range of abilities among men and women argues against prejudging the performance of any individual based on sex or sexual orientation alone.

4. William Beatty, "Gonadal Hormones and Sex Differences in Nonreproductive Behaviors," in *Sexual Differentiation*, vol. 11 of *Handbook of Behavioral Neurobiology*, ed. Arnold Gerall, Howard Moltz, and Ingeborg Ward (New York: Plenum Press, 1992).

5. Simon LeVay, *The Sexual Brain* (Cambridge: MIT Press, 1993), 101.

6. Cheryl McCormick, Sandra Witelson, and Edward Kingstone, "Left-handedness in Homosexual Men and Women: Neuroendocrine Implications," *Psychoneuroendocrinology* 15, no. 1 (1990): 69–76.

7. J. Lindesay, "Laterality Shift in Homosexual Men," *Neuropsychologia* 25 (1987): 965–69.

8. Unpublished results quoted in Dean Hamer and Peter Copeland, *The Science of Desire: The Search for the Gay Gene and the Biology of Behavior* (New York: Simon and Schuster, 1994).

9. Brian Gladue and William Beatty, "Sexual Orientation and Spatial Ability in Men and Women," *Psychobiology* 18, no. 1 (1990): 101–8.

10. Jay Hall and Doreen Kimura, "Sexual Orientation and Performance on Sexually Dimorphic Motor Tasks," *Archives of Sexual Behavior* 25, no. 4 (August 1995): 395–408.

11. Cheryl McCormick and Sandra Witelson, "Functional Cerebral Asymmetry and Sexual Orientation in Men and Women," *Behavioral Neuroscience* 108, no. 3 (June 1994): 525–32.

12. Laura Allen and Roger Gorski, "Sexual Orientation and the Size of the Anterior Commissure in the Human Brain," *Proceedings of the National Academy of Sciences of the U.S.A.* 89 (1992): 7199–7202.

13. A. Scamyougeras, S. F. Witelson, M. Bronskill, P. Stanchev, S. Black, G. Cheung, M. Steiner, and B. Buck, "Sexual Orientation and Anatomy of the Corpus Callosum," *Society for Neuroscience Abstracts* 20, no. 2 (1994): 1425.

14. The papers appear in the *Journal of Endocrinology* 40 (1968): 387–88, and 42 (1968): 163–64, respectively.

15. G. Dörner, T. Geierr, L. Ahrens, L. Krell, G. Münx, H. Sieler, E. Kittner, and H. Müller, "Prenatal Stress as Possible Etiologic Factor of Homosexuality of Human Males," *Endokrinology* 75 (1980): 365–86.

16. G. Dörner, B. Schenk, B. Schmiedel, and L. Ahrens, "Stressful Events in Prenatal Life of Bi- and Homosexual Men," *Experimental and Clinical Endocrinology* 81 (1983): 83–87.

17. V. Sigusch, E. Schorsch, M. Dannecker, and G. Schmidt, "Official Statement by the German Society for Sex Research on the Research of Prof. Dr.

Gunter Dörner on the Subject of Homosexuality," *Archives of Sexual Behavior* 11 (October 1983): 445–50.

18. Gunter Dörner, "Letter to the Editor," *Archives of Sexual Behavior* 12 (December 1983): 577–82.

19. Louis Gooren, "The Neuroendocrine Response of Luteinizing Hormone to Estrogen Administration in Heterosexual, Homosexual, and Transsexual Subjects," *Journal of Clinical Endocrinology and Metabolism* 63 (1986): 583–88.

20. Dörner, "Letter to the Editor," 577.

21. LeVay, *The Sexual Brain*, 126.

CHAPTER NINE   Sexual Genetics

1. Havelock Ellis and John Addington Symonds, *Sexual Inversion* (London, 1897; reprint, New York: Arno Press, 1975), 105. Hirschfeld cited in Franz Kallmann, "Comparative Twin Study on the Genetic Aspects of Male Homosexuality," *Journal of Nervous and Mental Disease* 115, no. 4 (1952): 283–98.

2. Ellis and Symonds, *Sexual Inversion*, 146.

3. Kallmann, "Comparative Twin Study."

4. Ibid., 283.

5. Alfred Kinsey, Wardell Pomeroy, and Clyde Martin, *Sexual Behavior in the Human Male* (Philadelphia: W. B. Saunders, 1948), iii.

6. Kallmann, "Comparative Twin Study," 297.

7. William Byne and Bruce Parsons, "Human Sexual Orientation: The Biologic Theories Reappraised," *Archives of General Psychiatry* 50, no. 3 (1993): 228–41.

8. J. Michael Bailey and Richard C. Pillard, "A Genetic Study of Male Sexual Orientation," *Archives of General Psychiatry* 48, no. 12 (1991): 1089–96.

9. J. Michael Bailey, Richard C. Pillard, Michael Neale, and Yvonne Agyei, "Heritable Factors Influence Sexual Orientation in Women," *Archives of General Psychiatry* 50, no. 3 (1993): 217–23.

10. Byne and Parsons, "Human Sexual Orientation."

11. Theodore Lidz, "Reply to 'A Genetic Study of Male Sexual Orientation,'" *Archives of General Psychiatry* 50, no. 3 (1993): 240.

12. See, for example, J. Michael Bailey and Deana S. Benishay, "Familial Aggregation of Female Sexual Orientation," *American Journal of Psychiatry* 150 (1993): 272–77, and Frederick Whitman, Milton Diamond, and James Martin, "Homosexual Orientation in Twins: A Report on Sixty-one Pairs and Three Triplet Sets," *Archives of Sexual Behavior* 22, no. 3 (1993): 187–206. See also Constance Holden, ed., "Random Samples," *Science* 268 (June 16, 1995): 1571.

13. Dean Hamer, Stella Hu, Victoria Magnuson, Nan Hu, and Angela Pattatucci, "A Linkage between DNA Markers on the X Chromosome and Male Sexual Orientation," *Science* 261 (July 16, 1993): 321–27.

14. Stella Hu, Angela Pattatucci, Chavis Patterson, David Fulker, Stacy

Cherny, Leonid Kruglyak, and Dean Hamer, "Linkage between Sexual Orientation and Chromosome Xq28 in Males but Not in Females," *Nature Genetics* 11 (November 1995): 248–56.

15. Jennifer Macke, Nan Hu, Stella Hu, Michael Bailey, Van King, Terry Brown, Dean Hamer, and Jeremy Nathans, "Sequence Variation in the Androgen Receptor Gene Is Not a Common Determinant of Male Sexual Orientation," *American Journal of Genetics* 53 (1993): 844–52.

CHAPTER TEN   Nature *and* Nurture

1. Robert Wesson, *Beyond Natural Selection* (Cambridge: MIT Press, 1991), 253.

2. Ibid., 142.

3. A more complete discussion of these concepts is Gerald M. Edelman, *Bright Light, Brilliant Fire, on the Matter of the Mind* (New York: Basic Books, 1992).

4. Wesson, *Beyond Natural Selection*, 263.

5. Ibid., 257.

6. June Reinisch and Stephanie Sanders, "Prenatal Hormonal Contributions to Sex Differences in Human Cognitive and Personality Development," in *Sexual Differentiation*, vol. 11 of *Handbook of Behavioral Neurobiology*, ed. Arnold Gerall, Howard Moltz, and Ingeborg Ward (New York: Plenum Press, 1992).

7. One is hard pressed to discover a book that has caused more unnecessary heartache and misery than Irving Bieber et al.'s *Homosexuality: A Psychoanalytic Study of Male Homosexuals* (New York: Basic Books, 1962), which purported to "prove" that parental behavior was at the root of male homosexuality (see chap. 15 of the present volume). For decades, parents were told to blame themselves for their children's homosexuality—causing cycles of blame and guilt and shame within families which tore many apart completely. The exhaustive 1970s studies of Bell and Weinberg concluded that "no particular phenomenon of family life can be singled out . . . as especially consequential for either homosexual or heterosexual development." See Alan Bell, Martin Weinberg, and Sue Hammersmith, *Sexual Preference: Its Development in Men and Women* (Bloomington: Indiana University Press, 1981), 191.

CHAPTER ELEVEN   Homosexual Identity Development

1. John Boswell, "Sexual and Ethical Categories in Pre-modern Europe," in *Homosexuality/Heterosexuality: Concepts of Sexual Orientation*, ed. David McWhirter, Stephanie Sanders, and June Reinisch (New York: Oxford University Press, 1990), 15.

2. Richard Isay, "Psychoanalytic Theory and the Therapy of Gay Men," in McWhirter, Sanders, and Reinisch, *Homosexuality/Heterosexuality*, 283.

3. Alan Bell, Martin Weinberg, and Sue Hammersmith, *Sexual Preference: Its Development in Men and Women* (Bloomington: Indiana University Press, 1981).

4. Richard R. Troiden, "The Formation of Homosexual Identities," *Journal of Homosexuality*, 17, nos. 1–2 (1989): 43–73.

5. John Reid, *The Best Little Boy in the World* (New York: Ballantine, 1973).

6. Vivian C. Cass, "Homosexual Identity Formation: A Theoretical Model," *Journal of Homosexuality* 4, no. 3 (1979): 219–35.

7. Ibid., 233.

8. Troiden, "Formation of Homosexual Identities," 54.

9. Gilbert Herdt, *Children of Horizons: How Gay and Lesbian Teens Are Leading a New Way Out of the Closet* (Boston: Beacon Press, 1993), 181.

10. Author's files.

11. Isay, "Psychoanalytic Theory," 295.

12. Cass, "Homosexual Identity Formation," 227.

13. Ibid., 220.

CHAPTER TWELVE   Stigma Management

1. Erving Goffman, *Stigma: Notes on the Management of Spoiled Identity* (Englewood Cliffs, N.J.: Prentice-Hall, 1963), 1.

2. Ibid., 2.

3. Ibid.

4. Richard R. Troiden, "The Formation of Homosexual Identities," *Journal of Homosexuality* 17, nos. 1–2 (1989): 43–73.

5. Gilbert Herdt, "Gay and Lesbian Youth," *Journal of Homosexuality* 17, nos. 1–2 (1989): 1–41.

6. Author's files.

7. For a more thorough discussion of this issue, see Carla Golden, "Diversity and Variability in Women's Sexual Identities," in *Lesbian Psychologies*, ed. the Boston Lesbian Psychologies Collective (Urbana: University of Illinois Press, 1987), 19–34.

8. Alan P. Bell and Martin S. Weinberg, *Homosexualities: A Study of Diversity among Men and Women* (New York: Simon and Schuster, 1978), and William Masters and Virginia Johnson, *Homosexuality in Perspective* (Boston: Little, Brown, 1979).

9. Richard C. Pillard, "The Kinsey Scale: Is It Familial?" in *Homosexuality/Heterosexuality: Concepts of Sexual Orientation*, ed. David McWhirter, Stephanie Sanders, and June Reinisch (New York: Oxford University Press, 1990), 88–114.

10. Golden, "Diversity and Variability," 25.

11. Although a comprehensive discussion of the complexities of lesbian identities is beyond the scope of this introductory book, several others are available which treat the issue in detail. An excellent beginning is *Lesbian Psychologies* (see note 7 above).

12. Gilbert Herdt, "Gay and Lesbian Youth, Emergent Identities, and Cultural Scenes at Home and Abroad," *Journal of Homosexuality* 22, nos. 3–4 (1991): 32.

13. See Leo Treadway and John Yoakam, "Creating a Safer School Environment for Lesbian and Gay Students," *Journal of School Health* 62, no. 7 (1992): 352–57.

14. An introduction to cultural variables in sexual orientation identity issues in Latinos, African Americans, Asian Americans, and Native Americans from a mental health perspective is Beverly Greene, "Ethnic-Minority Lesbians and Gay Men: Mental Health and Treatment Issues," *Journal of Consulting and Clinical Psychology* 62, no. 2 (1994): 243–51.

15. Alistair D. Williamson, "Is This the Right Time to Come Out?" *Harvard Business Review* (July-August 1993): 18–27.

16. Gordon Isaacs and Brian McKendrick, *Male Homosexuality in South Africa* (Capetown: Oxford University Press, 1992).

CHAPTER THIRTEEN　Bisexual and Transgender Identities

1. Alfred Kinsey, Wardell Pomeroy, and Clyde Martin, *Sexual Behavior in the Human Male* (Philadelphia: W. B. Saunders, 1948), 678, 639.

2. Sigmund Freud, "Analysis Terminable and Interminable" (originally written in English in 1937), *The Standard Edition of the Complete Psychological Works of Sigmund Freud*, vol. 23, ed. and trans. James Strachey (London: Hogarth, 1957), 216.

3. Fritz Klein, *Bisexualities: Theory and Research* (New York: Haworth, 1985).

4. J. Stokes, D. McKirnan, and R. Burzette, "Behavioral versus Self-labeling Definitions of Bisexuality: Implications for AIDS Risk," *International Conference on AIDS* 8, no. 2 (1992): abstract no. PoDD 5199.

5. Richard C. Pillard, "The Kinsey Scale: Is It Familial?" in *Homosexuality/ Heterosexuality: Concepts of Sexual Orientation*, ed. David McWhirter, Stephanie Sanders, and June Reinisch (New York: Oxford University Press, 1990), 88–114.

6. Margaret Nichols, "Lesbian Relationships: Implications for the Study of Sexuality and Gender," in McWhirter, Sanders, and Reinisch, *Homosexuality/ Heterosexuality*, 350–66.

7. Dolores Klaich, *Woman plus Woman* (Tallahassee: Naiad Press, 1989; reprint of *Woman + Woman*, New York: Morrow, 1974), 112.

8. M. Ross and J. Paul, "Beyond Gender: The Basis of Sexual Attraction in Bisexual Men and Women," *Psychological Reports* 71 (December 1992): 1283–90.

9. Jay Paul, "Bisexuality: Reassessing Our Paradigms of Sexuality," in *Two Lives to Lead: Bisexuality in Men and Women*, ed. Fritz Klein and Timothy Wolf (New York: Harrington Park Press, 1985), 30.

10. Peter Snyder, James Weinrich, and Richard Pillard, "Personality and Lipid Level Differences Associated with Homosexual and Bisexual Identity in Men," *Archives of Sexual Behavior* 23 (August 1994): 433–51.

11. George Brown, "A Review of Clinical Approaches to Gender Dysphoria," *Journal of Clinical Psychiatry* 51, no. 2 (1990): 57–64.

12. C. D. Doorn, J. Poortinga, and A. M. Verschoor, "Cross-Gender Identity in

Transvestites and Male Transsexuals," *Archives of Sexual Behavior* 23, no. 2 (1994): 185–201.

13. Modern surgical techniques and hormonal treatments make sexual reassignment possible to a substantial degree. In male-to-female transsexuals, the testicles are removed and scrotal skin used to construct "labia." The erectile tissue of the penis is removed and the penile skin inverted (like the finger of a glove) to line an artificial "vagina." Estrogen treatments produce breast enlargement and female body contours. Electrolysis removes facial and body hair. It is even possible to shave the throat cartilage surgically to reduce the Adam's apple. Because of the radical nature of the surgery, most male-to-female transsexuals lose the ability to experience orgasm.

In female-to-male transsexuals, hysterectomy (removal of the uterus and ovaries) and mastectomy (removal of breast tissue) are performed. Testosterone treatments lower the voice, increase muscle mass, and produce body hair. Various attempts to construct a "penis" surgically with tissue grafts have been tried, but none has been very successful. Many female-to-male transsexuals forgo this part of reassignment, satisfied with a clitoris grown larger by testosterone treatment. Although "penile" intercourse with a female is not possible, orgasm by other sexual techniques is.

14. H. Leif and L. Hubschman, "Orgasm in the Postoperative Transsexual," *Archives of Sexual Behavior* 22, no. 2 (1993): 145–57

15. P. Snaith, M. Tarsh, and R. Reid, "Sex Reassignment Surgery: A Study of 141 Dutch Transsexuals," *British Journal of Psychiatry* 163 (1993): 681–85.

16. E. Coleman, W. Bockting, and L. Gooren, "Homosexual and Bisexual Identity in Sex-Reassigned Female-to-Male Transsexuals," *Archives of Sexual Behavior* 22, no. 1 (1993): 37–50.

17. John Money, *Gay, Straight, and In-between: The Sexology of Erotic Orientation* (New York: Oxford University Press, 1988), 94.

18. Pedophilia, like tranvestophilia, is found almost exclusively in men and predominantly in men who are heterosexually oriented when they are limited to adult partners. There is no solid evidence that men who enjoy consensual, reciprocal sexual activities with adult men are any more subject to pedophilia or any paraphilia than men who are attracted to adult women. A recent study evaluated 352 victims of childhood sexual abuse to see if homosexuals were overrepresented in the group of perpetrators. They were not. The researchers concluded that "a child's risk of being molested by his or her [mother's] heterosexual partner is over 100 times greater than by someone who might be identifiable as being homosexual, lesbian or bisexual." See Carole Jenny, Thomas Roesler, and Kimberly Poyer, "Are Children at Risk for Sexual Abuse by Homosexuals?" *Pediatrics* 94, no. 1 (1994): 41–44.

19. Quoted in Hubert Kennedy, *Ulrichs: The Life and Works of Karl Heinrich Ulrichs* (Boston: Alyson, 1988), 61.

CHAPTER FOURTEEN From the Inquisition to the Holocaust

1. Quoted in John Boswell, *Christianity, Social Tolerance, and Homosexuality: Gay People in Western Europe from the Beginning of the Christian Era to the Fourteenth Century* (Chicago: University of Chicago Press, 1980), 120.

2. Malcolm Barber, *The New Knighthood: A History of the Order of the Temple* (Cambridge: Cambridge University Press, 1994).

3. Boswell, *Christianity, Social Tolerance, and Homosexuality*, 296.

4. Quoted in Malcolm Barber, *The Trial of the Templars* (Cambridge: Cambridge University Press, 1978), 45.

5. Colin Simpson, Lewis Chester, and David Leitch, *The Cleveland Street Affair* (Boston: Little, Brown, 1976).

6. Richard Ellman, *Oscar Wilde* (New York: Alfred A. Knopf, 1987).

7. Ibid., 418.

8. See Isabel Hull, *The Entourage of Kaiser Wilhelm II, 1888–1918* (Cambridge: Cambridge University Press, 1982).

9. Robert K. Massey, *Dreadnought: Britain, Germany, and the Coming of the Great War* (New York: Random House, 1991), 667.

10. Ibid., 123.

11. Ibid., 667.

12. Quoted in James Streakley, *The Homosexual Emancipation Movement in Germany* (Salem, N.H.: Ayer, 1975), 37.

13. Quoted in Hull, *Entourage of Kaiser Wilhelm II*, 238.

14. Quoted in Johannes Haller, *Philip Eulenburg: The Kaiser's Friend*, trans. Ethel Colburn Mayne (New York: Alfred A. Knopf, 1930).

15. George L. Mosse, *Nationalism and Sexuality, Respectability and Abnormal Sexuality in Modern Europe* (New York: Howard Fertig, 1985), 5.

16. J. Jennings Moss, "Good-bye Mr. Studds: The Nation's First Openly Gay Congressman Draws the Curtain on a Career of Breaking Ground Gracefully," *Advocate*, November 28, 1995.

17. Quoted in Richard Plant, *The Pink Triangle: The Nazi War against Homosexuals* (New York: Henry Holt, 1986). Unless otherwise noted, all quotations are taken from this source, currently the most comprehensive English language work on the Nazi persecution of homosexuals.

18. Ibid, 49.

19. The Communist Party's position statement on Paragraph 175 read: "In accordance with the scientific insights of modern times, the proletariat regards these relations as a special form of sexual gratification and demands the same freedom . . . for this form of sex life as for intercourse between the sexes." Streakley, *Homosexual Emancipation Movement*, 83.

20. Otto Weininger, *Sex and Character*, Authorized Translation from the Sixth German Edition (New York: G. P. Putnam's Sons, 1906).

21. For a discussion of the process of the appropriation of the German judiciary by the National Socialists during the Nazi era, see Ingo Müller, *Hitler's Justice: The Courts of the Third Reich* (Cambridge: Harvard University Press, 1991).

22. Heinz Heger, *The Men with the Pink Triangle* (Boston: Alyson, 1980), 22. This is an autobiographical account of the author's years in Nazi concentration camps.

23. Quoted in Streakley, *Homosexual Emancipation Movement*, 116.

24. Even today, the stories of homosexual Holocaust victims are in a sense suppressed. The two English-language books on the Nazi persecution of homosexuals are usually catalogued in American libraries among "gay and lesbian studies" and not among other works on the Holocaust. One must wonder why the systematic murder of homosexuals by the Nazis is thought to be about homosexuality rather than about systematic murder.

25. Müller, *Hitler's Justice*, 267.

26. Although heterosexual behavior such as oral-genital contact is usually also criminalized, "sodomy" laws are enforced almost exclusively against homosexuals. In the United States Supreme Court's *Bowers v. Hardwick* decision, upholding the state of Georgia's right to prosecute a man for a homosexual act discovered when a policeman barged into his bedroom, Justice White stated, "We express no opinion on the constitutionality of the Georgia statute as applied to other acts of sodomy." In several other states, acts classified as "sodomy" are illegal only between same-sex partners and not between opposite-sex partners.

27. In 1995, those states were Alabama, Arizona, Florida, Georgia, Idaho, Louisiana, Maryland, Massachusetts, Minnesota, Mississippi, Montana, North Carolina, Oklahoma, Rhode Island, South Carolina, Virginia, and Utah. Several states prohibit certain sex acts only between homosexual partners and do not criminalize the same acts between heterosexual partners; those states are Arkansas, Kansas, Missouri, Nevada, and Tennessee.

CHAPTER FIFTEEN   Salvation and Repair

1. The passages are Gen. 19:4–11, Lev. 18:22 and 20:13, 1 Cor. 6:9–10, 1 Tim. 1:9–10, and Rom. 1:26–27.

2. For a full discussion of this issue, see John Boswell, *Christianity, Social Tolerance, and Homosexuality: Gay People in Western Europe from the Beginning of the Christian Era to the Fourteenth Century* (Chicago: University of Chicago Press, 1980).

3. Exodus International, *An Introduction to Exodus International* (Exodus International, P.O. Box 2121, San Rafael, Calif., undated pamphlet).

4. Tim LaHaye, *What Everyone Should Know about Homosexuality* (Wheaton, Ill.: Living Books, Tyndale House Publishers, 1985), 31.

5. Bob Davies and Lori Rentzel, *Coming Out of Homosexuality: New Freedom for Men and Women* (Downers Grove, Ill.: Intervarsity Press, 1993), 33.

6. Ibid., 36.

7. Ibid., 101.

8. Ibid., 105.

9. Douglas Haldeman, "The Practice and Ethics of Sexual Orientation Conversion Therapy," *Journal of Consulting and Clinical Psychology* 62, no. 2 (1994): 221–27.

10. Ibid. See also "Rocky Mountain Low," *Advocate*, December 12, 1995, 12.

11. The film *One Nation under God* (Teodoro Maniaci and Francine Rzeznik, 3Z/Hourglass Productions) gives an excellent overview of ex-gay ministries. It includes the story of the cofounders of Exodus International, Gary Cooper and Robert Bussee, two "ex-gays" who discovered after several years of working together that they were in love with each other. These "ex" ex-gays appear on the jacket of the video version of the film in matching baby blue tuxedos, a picture taken at their ceremony of union.

12. Quoted in Michael Ybarra, "Going Straight: Christian Groups Press Gay People to Take a Heterosexual Path," *Wall Street Journal*, April 21, 1993.

13. Edmund Bergler, *Homosexuality: Disease or Way of Life?* (New York: Hill and Wang, 1956), 9.

14. Charles Socarides, Vamik Volkan, and Joseph Nicolosi, undated press release of the National Association for Research and Therapy of Homosexuality (NARTH), author's files.

15. Joseph Nicolosi, *Reparative Therapy of Male Homosexuality* (Northvale, N.J.: Jason Aronson, 1991) and *Healing Homosexuality: Case Studies of Reparative Therapy* (Northvale, N.J.: Jason Aronson, 1993).

16. Nicolosi, *Healing Homosexuality*, 211.

17. Ibid., 213.

18. Ibid., 193.

19. American Psychiatric Association, *Psychiatric News*, April 15, 1994, 18.

20. NARTH membership memo dated May 30, 1994, author's files.

21. Timothy Murphy, "Redirecting Sexual Orientation: Techniques and Justifications," *Journal of Sex Research* 29 (November 1992): 501–23.

22. Martin Sabshin, M.D., Press release of the American Psychiatric Association, May 1992.

23. Statement of Bryant Welch, American Psychological Association, January 26, 1990.

24. American Academy of Pediatrics Committee on Adolescence, *Pediatrics* 92 (1993): 631–33.

25. Charles Socarides, Harold Voth, C. Downing Tait, and Benjamin Kaufman, "AMA and Homosexuality" (letter to the editor), *Psychiatric News*, May 5, 1995, 23.

26. For the professional's perspective on reparative therapy, see Richard Isay, *Being Homosexual: Gay Men and Their Development* (New York: Farrar, Straus &

Giroux, 1989). Martin Duberman's *Cures* (New York: Dutton, 1991) is an autobiographical account of the author's many years of reorientation therapies of various types.

27. Socarides et al., "AMA and Homosexuality," 23.

CHAPTER SIXTEEN   Community and Power

1. San Francisco Lesbian and Gay History Project, "She Even Chewed Tobacco: A Pictorial Narrative of Passing Women in America," in *Hidden from History: Reclaiming the Gay and Lesbian Past*, ed. Martin Duberman, Martha Vicinus, and George Chauncey Jr. (New York: New American Books, 1989).

2. Originally published in the *Yearbook for Sexual Intermediates*, vol. 21, ed. Magnus Hirschfeld (1921), quoted in James Streakley, *The Homosexual Emancipation Movement in Germany* (Salem, N.H.: Ayer, 1975), 76.

3. Alan Stephenson, "The Homosexual: Another Untold Story: An Oral History of Bob Ruffing," quoted in John D'Emilio, *Sexual Politics, Sexual Communities: The Making of a Homosexual Minority in the United States, 1940–1970* (Chicago: University of Chicago Press, 1983), 26. The D'Emilio book is an excellent account of the rise and fall of the homophile movement.

4. D'Emilio, *Sexual Politics*, 28.

5. Ibid.

6. Donald Webster Cory, *The Homosexual in America*, quoted in D'Emilio, *Sexual Politics*, 33.

7. Quoted in D'Emilio, *Sexual Politics*, 65–66.

8. Chuck Rowland, quoted in Eric Marcus, *Making History: The Struggle for Gay and Lesbian Equal Rights, 1945–1990: An Oral History* (New York: HarperCollins, 1992), 34.

9. Chuck Rowland, quoted in D'Emilio, *Sexual Politics*, 71.

10. Rey Rivera, quoted in Marcus, *Making History*, 192.

11. Martha Shelly, quoted in Marcus, *Making History*, 180.

12. Quoted in D'Emilio, *Sexual Politics*, 232.

13. For an excellent discussion of the struggle between gay activists, the APA, and the Socarides group, see Ronald Bayer, *Homosexuality and American Psychiatry: The Politics of Diagnosis* (Princeton: Princeton University Press, 1987).

14. The most definitive account to date of the early years of the epidemic is Randy Shilts' comprehensive *And the Band Played On: Politics, People, and the AIDS Epidemic* (New York: Penguin, 1988).

15. Ibid., 312.

16. Ibid., 457.

17. Gary Remafedi, "Preventing the Sexual Transmission of AIDS during Adolescence," *Journal of Adolescent Health* 9, no. 2 (1989): 139–43.

18. John Gallagher, "A Fairy-tale Ending," *Advocate*, November 28, 1995, 25.

Summing Up

1. This phrase refers to the tale of a Chinese prince who rose from his lover's bed after a night of passion and discovered that the young man had fallen asleep on the sleeve of the prince's robe. Rather than disturb his lover's sleep, the prince cut the sleeve from the robe. See Bret Hinsch, *Passions of the Cut Sleeve: The Male Homosexual Tradition in China* (Berkeley: University of California Press, 1990).

2. Franklin Jones and Ronald Koshes, "Homosexuality and the Military," *American Journal of Psychiatry* 152, no. 1 (1995): 16–21.

Suggested Readings

In the past several years there has been an explosion of writings on the subject of homosexuality. The following is a very brief list of some of the excellent works on topics and ideas introduced in this book.

Sexual Histories

Boswell, John. *Christianity, Social Tolerance, and Homosexuality: Gay People in Western Europe from the Beginning of the Christian Era to the Fourteenth Century*. Chicago: University of Chicago Press, 1980. Scholarly and serious but a "must read" for those wanting to understand the development of Christian proscriptions of homosexual behavior.

Faderman, Lillian. *Surpassing the Love of Men: Romantic Friendship and Love between Women from the Renaissance to the Present*. New York: Quill, 1981. A lovely book that sensitively explores the rise and fall of "romantic friends."

Greenberg, David F. *The Construction of Homosexuality*. Chicago: University of Chicago Press, 1988. A comprehensive (over 600 pages) review of the history of homosexuality from a sociological perspective. An excellent reference book.

Kennedy, Hubert. *Ulrichs: The Life and Works of Karl Heinrich Ulrichs*. Boston: Alyson, 1988.

Miller, Neil. *Out of the Past: Gay and Lesbian History from 1869 to the Present*. New York: Vintage Books, 1995. An excellent overview of earlier gay and lesbian Americans.

Pomeroy, Wardell. *Dr. Kinsey and the Institute for Sex Research.* New York: Harper & Row, 1972. A terrific biography of a great scientist.

Sexual Biology

Hamer, Dean, and Peter Copeland. *The Science of Desire: The Search for the Gay Gene and the Biology of Behavior.* New York: Simon & Schuster, 1994.
LeVay, Simon. *The Sexual Brain.* Cambridge: MIT Press, 1993. A slim volume packed with information. The best discussion of the biological underpinnings of human sexual orientation written to date by the scientist who discovered one of them.
Money, John. *Gay, Straight, and In-between: The Sexology of Erotic Orientation.* New York: Oxford University Press, 1988. Somewhat technical and decidedly medical, but an excellent discussion of the science of defining and describing sexual behaviors.

Sexual Identities

Bell, Alan, Martin Weinberg, and Sue Hammersmith. *Sexual Preference: Its Development in Men and Women.* Bloomington: Indiana University Press, 1981. A bit dated now, but nonetheless a classic from the Kinsey Institute.
The Boston Lesbian Psychologies Collective, eds. *Lesbian Psychologies.* Urbana: University of Illinois Press, 1987. Explores many aspects of lesbian identities and relationships.
McWhirter, David, Stephanie Sanders, and June Reinisch, eds. *Homosexuality/Heterosexuality: Concepts of Sexual Orientation.* New York: Oxford University Press, 1990. Advanced reading for the most part, this book contains excellent reviews of developmental theories as well as other aspects of homosexuality by many leaders in their respective fields.

Sexual Politics

Bayer, Ronald. *Homosexuality and American Psychiatry: The Politics of Diagnosis.* Princeton: Princeton University Press, 1987. A dramatic account of the process by which homosexuality was deleted from the official diagnostic manual of the American Psychiatric Association.
D'Emilio, John. *Sexual Politics, Sexual Communities: The Making of a Homosexual Minority in the United States, 1940–1970.* Chicago: University of Chicago Press, 1983. An excellent account of the rise and fall of the homophile organizations and the dawn of the gay rights movement.
Duberman, Martin. *Cures.* New York: Dutton, 1991. An autobiographical account of the author's many years of reorientation therapies of various types.

Duberman, Martin, Martha Vicinus, and George Chauncey Jr., eds. *Hidden from History: Reclaiming the Gay and Lesbian Past.* New York: New American Library, 1989.

Ellman, Richard. *Oscar Wilde.* New York: Alfred A. Knopf, 1987. A superb recounting of an extraordinary life. Truly a book to be read and reread.

Marcus, Eric. *Making History: The Struggle for Gay and Lesbian Equal Rights, 1945–1990: An Oral History.* New York: HarperCollins, 1992. First-person accounts of activists and pioneers.

Plant, Richard. *The Pink Triangle: The Nazi War against Homosexuals.* New York: Henry Holt, 1986. The most comprehensive English-language work on the Nazi persecution of homosexuals.

Shilts, Randy. *And the Band Played On: Politics, People, and the AIDS Epidemic.* New York: Penguin, 1988. Another "must read." The story of discovery, courage, and folly in the beginnings of the AIDS epidemic.

Index

acquired immunodeficiency syndrome
(AIDS), 15, 176, 212, 240–44
Addams, Jane, 59
adolescence, 164–69, 176
AIDS. *See* acquired immunodeficiency
syndrome
Alexander the Great, 9
5-alpha-reductase deficiency, 107–8
Amazons, 13
ambiguous genitalia, 105–6
American Psychiatric Association
(APA), 94, 190–91, 195, 224, 227, 239
American Psychological Association,
229
amygdala, 115
androgen insensitivity syndrome, 105,
126, 144–45
andromemesis, 188
androphilia, 187
animals, "homosexuality" in, 111–13, 129
Anne I (queen of England), 53–54
anterior commissure, 128
anthropology, 4, 12–13, 15–18
anti-heterosexual bias, 174–75

anti-homosexual bias, 164, 170–78, 191,
193–95
APA. *See* American Psychiatric Association; American Psychological Association
Aquinas, Thomas, 23, 77, 97
Aristophanes, 9
ascertainment bias, 82, 117
Augustine, Saint, 52
aversive conditioning, 228

Bauman, Robert, 211
Benjamin, Harry, 184
berdache, 11–15, 99
Bergler, Edmund, 77, 223–25
Bieber, Irving, 94, 225, 239, 264n.7
biological correlates of sexual orientation: cerebral laterality, 122–23; and
genetics:—DNA studies, 141–46;
—twin studies, 137–41; hormonal,
106–8, 120–21, 132–33; neuroanatomi-
cal, 113–14, 128; and neuropsychology,
126–27; summary, 156–57
birth control, 22, 26, 50

LIBRARY OF CONGRESS CATALOGING-IN-PUBLICATION DATA

Mondimore, Francis Mark, 1953–
    A natural history of homosexuality / Francis Mark Mondimore.
      p.   cm.
    Includes bibliographical references and index.
    ISBN 0-8018-5349-4 (alk. paper). — ISBN 0-8018-5440-7 (pbk. :
alk. paper)
    1. Homosexuality.   2. Sex (Biology)
HQ76.25.M649   1996
306.76'6—dc20   96-16191